Fighting for the Soul of General Practice

The Algorithm Will See You Now

T0200255

Global Health Humanities

Series Editors: Susan Hogan and Anna Greenwood

Print ISSN: 2752-8545 | **Online ISSN:** 2752-8553

Global Health Humanities is a new Intellect book series that examines the health humanities from a number of perspectives, incorporating: medical humanities; health humanities; history of medicine; and arts and health. Contributions to the series focus on a wide range of subjects and utilise numerous methodologies and perspectives.

The series has multiple formats: traditional scholarly monographs; edited collections; and shorter format volumes. Authors include established scholars in the field, emerging early-career scholars, and practitioners. The series will appeal to health humanities scholars; clinicians and carers; and arts and humanities practitioners, as well as the learned general public.

In this series:

Fighting for the Soul of General Practice

The Algorithm Will See You Now

Rupal Shah and Jens Foell

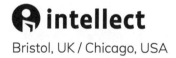

Bristol, UK / Chicago, USA

First published in the UK in 2023 by
Intellect, The Mill, Parnall Road, Fishponds, Bristol, BS16 3JG, UK

First published in the USA in 2023 by
Intellect, The University of Chicago Press, 1427 E. 60th Street, Chicago,
IL 60637, USA

A catalogue record for this book is available from the British Library.

Copy editor: MPS Limited
Cover designer: Tanya Montefusco
Production editor: Debora Nicosia
Cover image: Jens Foell, *There Is No NHS*, 2021.

Paperback ISBN 978-1-78938-839-8
ePDF ISBN 978-1-78938-840-4
ePUB ISBN 978-1-78938-841-1

Part of the Global Health Humanities series
Print ISSN 2752-8545
Online ISSN 2752-8553

Printed and bound by CPI Group (UK) Ltd, Croydon CR0 4YY

Index by Lyn Greenwood

To find out about all our publications, please visit our website.
There you can subscribe to our e-newsletter, browse or download our
current catalogue, and buy any titles that are in print.

www.intellectbooks.com

This is a peer-reviewed publication.

Contents

'This is an honest dispatch from the frontlines of the conflict between industrializing bureaucracies and the ongoing care of each person. It is a hopeful song for clinicians who, when the algorithm says no, breach the protocol and go the extra mile for each patient.'
Victor M. Montori
Professor of Medicine, Mayo Clinic, Rochester, US

'UK general practice is at a precarious crossroads. This book captures the essence of traditional, relationship-based, family doctor care, which is now under threat from a number of forces – not least the technologization of medicine and the inexorable encroachment of algorithmic, if-then decision-making on relational and narrative-based clinical method. Shah and Foell have documented the essence of what we risk losing. Perhaps, if their warnings are heeded, they will also succeed in retaining and restoring what they rightly describe as general practice's "soul".'
Trish Greenhalgh
Professor of Primary Care Health Sciences, University of Oxford, UK

'This is 21st-century general practice, observed from within a dysfunctional NHS that has been deliberately starved of resources over more than a decade; yet it will make you fall back in love with what the job and the service has been, should be and still could be with a little more trust and understanding from those in power.'
Iona Heath
Former president of the Royal College of General Practitioners, UK

'A rich, wonderful, profound and moving book. I was immersed in the many stories and heartfelt, sometimes harrowing, observations. The need to innovatively transform health and social care, and particularly mental health care, by integrating the work of primary care with social care, local councils, voluntary sectors, communities, patients and families is now vital. Written in an authentic and deeply compassionate way, *Fighting for the Soul of General Practice* provides a broad and comprehensive understanding of the issues and challenges we face.'
Michael West
Professor of Organizational Psychology, Lancaster University Management School, UK

Figures

Acknowledgements

Rupal
This book came into being over the course of several years and is
an expression of what being a general practitioner (GP) has meant
to me over a couple of decades of practice, and an articulation of
the forces that are unravelling our profession. It involved Jens
and I taking large chunks of our spare time to formulate our ideas,
write, and talk to one another. As we are both practising GPs,
much of this time was carved out from evenings and weekends.
The last chapter is called 'A Labour of Love', and that's what this
has been. We would like to thank our families for their support
and to apologize for being absent. I would like to dedicate it to my
beautiful daughters, Ava and Anya, and to my husband Alistair.
I would like to thank friends for spending their time reading draft
versions and for giving me their feedback: John Spicer, John
Launer, Miriam, Caryn, Cathy, Veena, Sarah, and my wonderful
book club. Thanks also to our amazing practice team, my patients,
and Vayu for introducing me to Intellect publishers. I would
particularly like to mention Anna Greenwood, the series editor, for
being responsive, insightful, and patient.

Jens
I am grateful for the relationships that made a collection of stories
turn into a book. To name a few, there are John Launer and the
network of narrative practitioners. There are Jonathon Tomlinson
and Deborah Swinglehurst. Sheepishly, I can promise my wife
Esyllt that book-related screen time will diminish now. My children
Mali and Efan have been my fiercest critics, whether it relates to
adherence to the theme 'power, bureaucracy, vibes and the symbolic
order' or to errors of syntax. My colleague Martin has the gift of
listening. I owe thanks to the porters, domestics, and healthcare
assistants in hospital and to the receptionists in our practice, whose
work is underappreciated. And of course, I must name the creators
of the countless absurd e-mails and directives that remind me every
day of the necessity of enshrining their activities in stories.

Prologue

Jens
I am writing this prologue in a six-bed bay inhabited by six men in a surgical ward in a hospital in North Wales, waiting for an operation to repair my leg. The surgery has been delayed several times. Four patients have dementia, one has end-stage cancer. We're all waiting for our time to be processed; time for an operation, time to be discharged. The days are long. We are observing the ritual of the medical drama unfolding. It feels like being part of a sitcom or doing a stint of participant observation in the late stages of a crumbling NHS. Outside there are ten ambulances waiting and the local health board has issued a major emergency over the Christmas period.

I moved to the United Kingdom after studying medicine in Germany and obtaining a postgraduate qualification in rehabilitation medicine. I thought the NHS could be a lever to achieve inclusivity. GP training in the United Kingdom taught me about relational medicine and the role of relationships in healing. As my recent enforced personal experience of being a patient demonstrates: the NHS runs on goodwill!

This book started life as a collection of unrelated miniature docu-dramas written by Rupal and me. They are vignettes which focus on the predicaments that practising GPs face in their everyday work, including dilemmas about rationing and decisions relating to deservedness and entitlement in the context of chronic underfunding and bureaucracy. Which brings me back to the bay in the Welsh hospital, where I see first-hand how scarcity affects care. It means long delays. It means no resources and a fight for the very little that is left. Even within this strained context, many, many people go the extra mile, as I have experienced in my own journey, which has not yet come to an end.

Rupal
As well as working as a GP for the past twenty years, I have been involved in education for a large part of my career. When I talk

to trainee doctors about emotional engagement, attention, and compassion-recurring themes in this book, I notice that I am increasingly met with disengagement, dissatisfaction, and disenchantment, both within general practice and within hospital settings. Perhaps this explains the inexorable exodus of doctors and nurses from the NHS. As hard as we try, we struggle to retain people and despite NHS mission statements about valuing staff, burnout abounds. Based on my personal experience and on the conversations I have had with trainees and colleagues, my sense is that burnout emanates not only from working within scarcity. It is also linked to moral injury – continually behaving in a way that is in conflict with our values, and with no agency or prospect of changing things. Healthcare systems are there to make people feel better and live longer but can instead turn out to be anonymous, generic, brutalizing, and cruel. The goodwill that Jens describes and on which the system depends is generated when people feel connected to one another and when there are trusting relationships in the workplace which allow staff to use discretion and their own judgement when the situation demands it, rather than uncritically following guidelines and protocol. Acting upon goodwill is an antidote to moral injury.

In our book, we use themes we have encountered in our own professional practice to illustrate and explore these issues within a GP context. The stories are amalgams of experiences I have had with patients rather than describing real encounters. 'Ed and Lily' who feature in 'Pigeonholes' and in 'Passports for Passing' are the exceptions and I am grateful to Ed for letting me tell their story. To practise as a GP is a huge privilege, one which has allowed Jens and me to be immersed in the lives of our patients and in our communities for the past two decades. It is not a job which should ever become solely technical and transactional. I hope we describe why in the chapters that follow and offer an alternative view.

Introduction: Standardising General Practice

His blood sugar readings were spectacularly high. Because of this, he was losing weight, passing too much urine, more thirsty than normal. He needed insulin.

But insulin needs to be stored in a fridge. He couldn't manage it because his wife had thrown him out and he was sleeping in his car, which was in our car park, to avoid parking tickets. This was an unofficial arrangement. The official answer would have been 'no'.

But there he was, in our car park in his Ford Mondeo. At that time, he needed to see the practice nurses regularly because he had a wound on his arm from a fight that had to be dressed – and he took the opportunity to use our toilet to have a wash when he came in. We turned a blind eye.

He was in a bad way. He asked if he could store his insulin in our practice fridge.

Also, he was hungry. He asked if he could have a bit of food, maybe a loaf of bread. We have supplies in our kitchen for the practice staff.

It was getting intrusive now. We were starting to think, 'We can't help him this much, not in this way. We can't make exceptions. There are ways to behave, there are rules, and he is making us break them. There are other services set up to help him, social services, food banks, hostels, we have given him phone numbers, made referrals. We've already done all that can be expected of us.'

So, he drove off in his Ford Mondeo and we didn't see him again.

Looking Through Rose-Tinted Glasses

The archetypal general practitioner (GP) who lived in a pre-digital, pre-bureaucratic era has been portrayed in numerous books, films, and paintings. Such images evoke a certain idealized memory of the GP figure who lurks in the background of our collective imagination.[1] The one who knows the family, the one who will go out for home visits, the one with the long-standing patient relationships made up of many brief encounters. An individual who will give personalized care, instead of generic advice that could apply to anyone. In Jens's practice, a print of Norman Rockwell's 'Doctor and Doll'[2] portrays an old-fashioned doctor indulgently examining the doll of a young girl, surrounded by accoutrements signifying his privilege. It serves as an heirloom and captures this tradition of General Practice.

Medical students and GP trainees are sometimes asked to read about the real-life archetypal single-handed GP, John Eskell who devoted his life to serving his patients and who was depicted in John Berger's classic 1967 photodocumentary book, *A Fortunate Man* under the pseudonym John Sassall.[3] However, it is less well known that Eskell took his own life in the end. The exact circumstances are unknown, but the intensity of his dedication to work is glorified in the book.

What does this mean for us now? This archetypal GP can and should no longer exist. The context has changed – society has moved on and the fault lines underlying the deceptively benign surface of the archetype have been exposed. The old-fashioned family doctor's perceived omnipresence was often at the expense of family, burnt out and sometimes dubious practices which neither patients nor the state had sufficient agency to challenge. Besides, the era in which the spouse of a GP unobtrusively smoothed his way

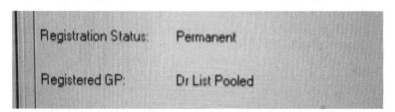

FIGURE I.1: The generic 'Dr. List Pooled', screenshot from a computerized GP record. It signifies that the patient has no named GP, but is instead part of a generic, pooled list of patients registered with the practice rather than with an individual. Jens Foell, 2021.

(as Eskell's wife did) by acting as an unofficial or, often, official practice manager, secretary, and household administrator has passed. The same applies to the matron as nursing equivalent, who had no husband and no family and could dedicate herself completely to service.

This book is not about nostalgia, and we are not suggesting a return to a 'better' time. It is not that as practising GPs, Jens and I object to being embedded within and accountable to the systems we are part of. But we do want to consider how, and with what, the gap left by the archetypal GP has been filled. We use anonymized stories, in which demographic details have been altered, to describe the effect of different facets of bureaucracy on our ability to build relationships with patients and to maintain a nuanced, individualized approach to each encounter. We explore the prominence and effect of protocol – by which we mean official procedures and rules. Jens and I are interested in the way professional relationships are influenced by protocol: between and within organizations; and most importantly with patients/clients/ service users – the people we are there to serve.

An aspect of bureaucracy which this book will revisit time and again is the detachment, autonomy, and often silent dominance of bureaucratic processes. In the context of digitalization of the workplace, they are enshrined and reified in computerized algorithms which lay out treatment pathways and referral guidelines. In the context of governance, they manifest as time and manpower-consuming audits and checklists.

Bureaucracy
Bureaucracy (n.): 'government by bureaus', especially 'tyrannical officialdom'. [...] [F]rom French *bureaucratie* [...] *bureau* 'office', literally 'desk' [and the] Greek suffix -*kratia* denoting 'power of' (*Online etymological dictionary*).

Bureaucracy exists as a safeguard against injustice and exploitation by those with power. But it doesn't have pleasant associations for most people – anonymity, frustration, futility, and fighting – wrestling with paperwork, drowning in red tape, and battling officious staff who take pleasure in exercising their power. It is not a word associated with relationships, health, or healing.

3

Yet, as practising GPs, Jens and I are street-level bureaucrats.
Lipsky first coined the term 'street-level-bureaucrat' in
1980, which he used to link occupations as diverse as law and
social work.[4] He proposed that all these professions had a
commonality in that they are organized as regulated systems in
which workers negotiate the needs of the client with the agenda
of the organization. The inherent paradox is that all clients are to
be treated equally while at the same time the professional should
be responsive to the individual. 'Street-level' implies a distance
from central decision-making. This phenomenon has become ever
more prominent within society as a whole and applies specifically
to public sector workers in health (primary and secondary care),
education, housing, and social care; where there are protocols to
be adhered to and defined outputs to achieve, while at the same
time trying to accommodate the individual needs of patients,
students, and service users. Jens and I have been GPs for most of
our professional lives and can only draw on our own experiences
to illustrate these themes – so like us, our book is situated in
primary care. However, we suspect that much of what we write
will resonate with people from other spheres of life, not just public
sector organizations but also the commercial sector – we are all
accustomed nowadays to automated telephone lines, chatbots,
unhelpful website FAQs, the frustration of being unable to connect
with another human being who will listen to our *particular*
question and give us something other than a generic, off-the-
peg answer. The same issues that are facing society at large have
changed the way in which we work as GPs and the care we give.

NHS GPs are part of a highly protocolized, complex
organization whose rules and structures we have no choice but to
respect, both from a governance point of view and also to prevent
us from becoming alienated within our own profession. We are
obliged to support the mission statements of our organizations.
We work within the NHS and are bound by its codes of practice. As
a profession, we are woven into the social fabric and landscape of
our practice populations, but we spend much of our time filling in
templates with pre-structured digitalized interfaces.

There are good reasons for public sector organizations,
including NHS England, to have standardized approaches and
targets and outcome measures to demonstrate standards being
achieved and value for money. The legitimacy conferred by the

State on the medical profession is essential to our existence in the United Kingdom, as it is worldwide.[5] However, there are inadvertent consequences on the nature of the relationship between clinician and patient, arising from an altered conception of professional identity and purpose, which we discuss below.

Aspects of Bureaucracy Which Impact Relational Care
Regulation and Control

There has been a substantial move towards standardization in the last few decades. This impacts everything that GPs do – from the drugs we prescribe, and the referral pathways available to us, to the accessibility standards of the surgery building and hygiene standards (no more toys in the waiting room for us, even pre-COVID-19). Hand-in-hand with this, there comes the need for regulation, accelerated by high-profile cases such as Harold Shipman, the infamous GP serial killer who is estimated to have killed 250 victims during his career.

At an organizational level, the Care Quality Commission (CQC) checks that GP services in the UK provide 'safe, effective, and high-quality care', through a process of regular inspections. The CQC is a public sector organization which reports to the Department of Health and Social Care. It was created in 2009. It is an amalgamation of three pre-existing state-run regulatory bodies but has eclipsed its predecessors in terms of prominence, influence, and importance. CQC inspections can take place every five years (more often for surgeries not rated 'Good' or 'Outstanding') and involve working through a laborious checklist that must be ticked off each time.

CQC checks are representative of the overall culture of the NHS at this point in its history. When something goes wrong, the likelihood is that the checklists expand further. It is a huge industry. It is not certain whether the inspections really do drive up quality of care, or if they are there for their own sake now, having acquired an independent life of their own and a societal standing which can no longer be challenged. It is expensive to satisfy the demands of the checklists – in monetary terms and in terms of the finite resources of time, manpower, and energy.

As well as organizational regulation, at an individual level, the behaviour of doctors can come under scrutiny from our own regulatory body, the General Medical Council (GMC). Cases such as Harold Shipman accelerated the implementation of changes designed to safeguard patients. The looming menace of the GMC figures

5

prominently in the collective consciousness of doctors. There are many stories of investigations dragging on for years, leaving a stain on professional reputation and emotions that can't be washed out. The risk of breaking rules, explicit or implicit, lingers pervasively, an ominous shadow that permeates our decision-making. It's important to stay in the pack and not be cast out. In medicolegal terms, it is called the 'Bolitho principle' – what would others in our profession do in the same situation?[6] If we have acted in the same way as most of our peers would **and** if there is an understandable basis for the decision, we are safe. The Bolitho principle theoretically recognizes that applying professional judgement is not synonymous with applying the evidence base; except that now, what constitutes 'normal' behaviour *is* to adhere to protocol and guidelines. There has been a significant cultural shift in the past two decades, coinciding with the advent of what has been termed the 'scientific bureaucratic method', whereby the discretion afforded to clinicians about when and how to apply evidence-based medicine for the benefit of their individual patients has been eroded. The new normal is to follow rules.[7,8]

The rules apply not only to approaches to treatment but also to relationships, the effects of which we expand on in the chapters entitled 'Weaponized Bureaucracy' and 'Pigeonholes'. The change in culture which has arisen as a result of our focus on regulation and protocol has had the inadvertent effect of creating boundaries between doctor and patient, which doctors are careful to maintain in order to avoid putting our heads above the parapet and drawing attention to our practice. So, it is not OK any more to form friendships with patients in the way that once was commonplace – relationships must be clearly defined. This is not explicitly written down but is outside of 'normal' practice, deviation from which at the very least would generate unspoken questions from colleagues. Giving out details, like a personal telephone number or e-mail address, is also not a neutral act. The other members of the practice team might raise concerns over such special treatment. What happens when Dr. Phone-number-giver is away, who is going to step in? Why should only a few, selected patients (the 'poppets' as they were termed in a qualitative research paper) get enhanced access to their GP? What gives us the right to pick our favourites?[9] This is the balancing act: equity vs. personal holding work; autonomy vs. standardized practice.[10]

In a culture where professional boundaries are important and there are standardized conceptions of professional demeanour, there is a degree of 'emotional labour' required by practitioners to maintain the obligatory facade of calm, sympathetic detachment, which is often in conflict with their inner feelings.[11] This may be reflected in the language of the consultation, which can be deliberately impersonal and therefore can inadvertently create distance.[12,13] You may have heard your GP or another clinician you have seen in the practice using phrases such as *'we* would recommend you ... (take a pill, are referred, exercise more often, eat less ...)'. Who is this enigmatic, aloof 'we'? The answer is that 'we' refers to the system and this choice of language signifies the reluctance of clinicians to be exposed as emotional individuals.[14]

Structural Change

The old-fashioned, archetypal GP was probably single-handed, based within his own home, with his wife or secretary taking care of the small amount of associated administrative work – these family doctors were often professionally situated within their own families. It sounds idyllic, but the truth was different. Like being a parent, a GP could never clock off from his responsibility for his patients. The 1950 Collings Report analyzed the quality of general practice at the time and described poor standards of care and inadequate working conditions, with doctors reporting high levels of stress, isolation, and lack of support.[15] However, it wasn't until the late 1960s that group practices became more common, and GPs started to leave home to work in health centres.

The landscape of General Practice now would be unrecognizable to the Doctor with the Doll. The increased prominence of regulation and standardization has coincided with GPs being incorporated into large multi-professional primary care teams comprising a variety of clinicians (e.g., nurses, pharmacists, social prescribers, physiotherapists, paramedics, health coaches, and physician's associates) who may work from different locations with different professional cultures and who may not know one another personally. Technology is being used to ever greater effect. Consultations are now often remote and continuity of care with the same doctor has become less common. This has changed the nature of relationships within teams and with patients. In parallel with developments in the food retail sector, the family doctor as corner-shop has become part of a wider network. The organizations have become more complex and are often located in purpose-built premises, leaving the family atmosphere of the now obsolete corner-shop era behind. Your local GP surgery is like an 'NHS local', a peripheral outlet of bigger health providers. These local outlets now collaborate in serving the populations as primary care networks.

The family atmosphere is also disrupted by clinicians' own families. Healthcare professionals are now allowed to have lives. They must successfully negotiate their professional and personal care commitments. Work-life balance has become a hotly debated issue and the fear of burning out has increased. Working part-time has been the answer for many, but working part-time means that continuity of care is more difficult to achieve. 'Portfolio GP' is the term used for GPs who have multiple, fragmented work commitments and applies to both of us – as well as being GPs, Jens and I have educational roles and Jens works as an advisor for the National Institute for Clinical Excellence (NICE).

Access has changed too, accelerated by the COVID-19 pandemic. The queues of patients outside the surgery, waiting to be seen, have shortened or disappeared. But queues always re-emerge somewhere when demand outstrips supply. Instead, they have moved either to endless telephone loops ('If you want to hear your blood test result, PRESS 2') or to the queue of e-mails waiting to be opened. It is now a contractual obligation for GP practices to provide some sort of web-based triage system, whereby patients fill in a form online to describe their symptoms. In Out-of-Hours care, an invisible Hogwarts sorting hat in the form of an algorithm that is enacted by call handlers directs people to a range of options, from self-care to the local pharmacy or A&E – or failing that to the GP practice itself to deal with and respond to as it feels appropriate (text message, telephone call, video call, or face-to-face consultation). Emergency services and Out-of-Hours care step in as overflow services for unmet needs.

The form on which patients make their case for being seen by a clinician aims to provide a more standardized gateway to care than is achieved by negotiating with reception staff. However, a form doesn't lend itself to nuance; and algorithms don't understand ambiguity, so when they are used to establish the truth, meaning can be missed. Feeling unwell isn't always so easy to describe to a computer. A person with depression which is causing headaches may find themselves receiving a text message from their GP advising rest and paracetamol, or they will receive a recommendation to go immediately to A&E, even if they know for sure that this will be a waste of time for everybody. So, they are forced to reformulate their story to eventually get access to where they want to be seen – they must try again to negotiate with the algorithm, or perhaps they will give up. Computer says 'No'.

In a time of such rapid change to the structure and form of clinical practice, there has been no unifying vision of how to balance the conflict generated by competing, sometimes irreconcilable forces. Each new measure is introduced piecemeal without consideration of how it affects other aspects of the service. There hasn't been a coherent approach to implementing governance and quality assurance processes with reference to the bigger picture of balancing risk within complexity, maintaining relationships and finding meaning for patients within the consultation. We have gone from shabby corner-shops to shiny new supermarkets which look impressive but where the electrics are faulty and where brand is key. We are selling a vision which we can't deliver.

It's All About the Output

The quality and outcomes framework was introduced within the new GP contract of 2004 and catalyzed template-driven chronic disease management, whereby payment is attached to performance across a range of clinical indicators (diabetes control, blood pressure management, etc.). There are also a multiplicity of other incentive schemes in existence, which reward practices that achieve immunization targets, perform enough cervical smears, and undertake the right number of structured medication reviews. The list goes on and on. Practices that do badly end up financially unviable, as well as being flagged up by regulators as poorly performing. However, data about hard outcomes like gains in life expectancy and softer outcomes like quality of life are not easy to interpret – it is impossible to attribute multifactorial variables like life expectancy and quality of life to single interventions in the presence of so many confounding factors.

This protocol-driven medicine could be said to replace the patient's narrative with an algorithm – from stories to data, then to meta-data. It promotes prioritization of provider-organization-driven proactive activity, meaning that healthcare workers commonly face a conflict of interest between listening to the patient or listening to the demands of surveillance medicine for data (in the form of measurements such as blood pressure, smoking status, and cholesterol). An unintended consequence of template-driven chronic disease management is that continuity of care within primary care teams has become more difficult to achieve. Many patients have had to get used to navigating a disrupted parkour of appointments through the maze of the extended primary healthcare team. In contrast, patients, particularly those who are frail and vulnerable long for personalized care and a trusted relationship that can tailor the targets of population health to their individual needs; or for a clinician to act as a trusted confidante and travel agent in the journey through healthcare systems. There is an abundance of evidence to show that patients are right to want this type of care and that continuity of care and a strong therapeutic alliance improves outcomes.[16,17]

The emergence of targets, referral pathways and disease algorithms have parallels with the automatization of labour in industrial mass production, which relies on breaking down work processes into small component parts. The aim is to achieve complexity reduction: break a complicated process down into parts and distribute them, like using a manual to build a large Lego structure. This has meant that we now work in a system that tries to measure what we do by outputs such as the number of people with high blood pressure who are treated to target; or the number of people with diabetes who have well-controlled blood sugars; or our compliance with prescribing targets; or the number of care-plans we generate for people with complex, chronic disease. Governance, managed care, and the correct form of 'patient-centredness' now structure the space of uncertainty. Any decision taken in this space of uncertainty is formatted and enacted within bureaucratic processes, with the background hum of demands which are coming in constantly, via text messages, e-mails, computer screen messages, and computerized practice notes. A factory with an endless quota of outcomes to manufacture. The daily grind. General Practice combines the challenges of industrial and post-industrial working practices. Whilst manufacturing relies on breaking down complex work processes into standardized components (Fordism), post-industrial information management transforms these practices into a digital world (see Figure I.2).

'The general practice of our post-millennial era is modelled increasingly on a "Sort, Fix or Send" (SFS) model'.[18] SFS implies that patients should be triaged, treated for the defined problem with which they initially presented, or referred to a different service. It

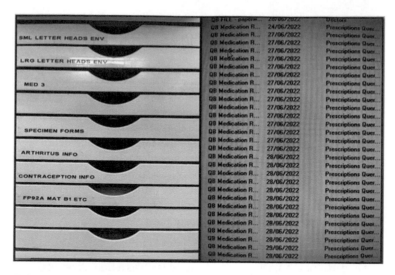

FIGURE I.2: Analogue and digital filing systems are in parallel use in primary care. Jens Foell, 2021.

is a natural result of working in a system which relies so heavily on measurable outputs. The approach suits systems which are geared towards measuring, recording, and producing defined outputs. It works fine as a way to manage problems which can be treated as discrete episodes – for example, acute appendicitis; or a heart attack; or a fractured femur. Unfortunately, though, most of what we deal with as GPs is not comprised of such defined illness; much of our work doesn't and shouldn't fit into neat boxes. We live within the daily soap opera of lives and families, where the meaning and lived experience of illness is as important as diagnosis and treatment.[19,20] The SFS approach is especially problematic when applied to mental health, social care and safeguarding, to ageing and terminal care – which we expand on later in the book. It is antithetical to establishing the personal relationships enjoyed by the Doctor with the Doll.

The methods of GP work: thinking, feeling, knowing, organizing, using imagination, detective work, holding work, and emotional engagement are not like constructing a piece of Lego. The allure of decontextualized knowledge with its reliance on numbers can turn out to be invidious when applied indiscriminately in the swampy lowlands of primary care.[21,22] General Practice deals with intractable situations, with people who have been discharged from secondary care services, and people with disabilities who are difficult to fit into the neatly defined access criteria of services designed for diseases. It takes on the tasks of helping the ones that cannot be helped and holding the ones that cannot be held. This is a huge component of the workload. End-of-life care and frailty care predominantly take place in the community – a *good* death should be the measure of the quality of service delivered. However, the factors that support a good death – pastoral care in challenging times, emotional availability and on-going care for the wider family or community – are difficult to measure.

In hospital medicine, there are at least some measurable outputs – people being discharged home; operations being carried out; death in hospital. The death of a patient is an endpoint. However, in primary care, where the lives of caregivers, family, and the community go on, it is only the end of a chapter. Encounters within relationships do not end in a neatly packaged final output such as a final diagnosis or curative treatment that ends all ills – they return unexpectedly in different guises and at different times. General Practice life is not linear. It is circular and the circular loops are not predictable. It is messy and confusing, like the storyline in a soap opera.

In the film *Modern Times*, Charlie Chaplin portrayed the alienation induced by industrial manufacturing processes. The worker eventually disappears into the machinery. Similarly, we risk conflating the bureaucratic processes which govern us with patient care and ultimately disappearing into the protocol.

Decision-Making in Real Life

The changes to healthcare described above have implications for clinical decision-making, illustrated in the case below. The trains of thought running through the mind of the clinician must be compressed into a single track by the end of the consultation, which anachronistically, is still only ten minutes long for most GPs.

He wheeled himself into my room, manoeuvring himself skilfully through the narrow doorway.

He brought a smell into the room of stale alcohol, old sweat, and clothes which were put away when they were still wet.

His beard was matted and grey, unlike his scalp which was smooth and hair free.

I wanted to talk to him about his diabetes and hence remove, Pac-man style, some of the yellow triangles appearing on his screen which indicated everything that needed to be done to get him to target. His sugar control was still terrible, despite all the complications he had developed because of his diabetes – like his above knee amputation for instance.

But he cut me off mid-flow, 'All I want is some Viagra, doc. How much can you give me?'

'What do you need Viagra for?'

I meant, 'What do you need Viagra for?'

How could he respond to this? Maybe a quick biology lesson? It was just as well for me that he chose not to expose my italicised you.

'It's for the hooker who comes over. I need a bit of help these days.' He winked at me, enjoying my discomfort, getting his revenge. 'If it costs too much, I'm willing to swap my statin for it. Honestly, I couldn't give a **** about my cholesterol.'

A train of thought – The bureaucratic track

'What do you need Viagra for?' stands for 'Why do you want to talk about sex when the important thing here is your diabetes, which is the reason you need the Viagra in the first place? Look at everything that we have to tackle – nothing is going well. Your sugar levels are through the roof, your blood pressure is too high, you've just told me you're not taking your statin so your cholesterol is doing its own thing. Your diabetes is going to kill you early and it's also ruining our practice achievement targets.'

Another train of thought – The guideline track

'What do you need Viagra for', 'And do you use condoms? Unprotected sex is dangerous you know. I can offer you screening for sexually transmitted infections or show you how to book an appointment at the local GU clinic. And another thing, do you suffer from chest pains? Viagra isn't safe if you get angina [...]. Hmmm [...] well ok the guideline says I can give you up to four Viagra tablets a month on the NHS [...] but no, you are not allowed to swap your statin for any more than that.'

Another train of thought – The medicolegal track

I am not sure if I can prescribe Viagra for you if you're not in a 'stable' relationship. How old is the prostitute you see? She might be vulnerable. Is she being trafficked? How can she consent to having sex with you anyway? Having sex with prostitutes can lead to serious sexually transmitted infections. What does the GMC have to say about this? Am I going to get in trouble? By prescribing, I am causing you and her potential harm, I won't do it.

Another train of thought – The relational track

You are probably very lonely. Why shouldn't you get some pleasure and why am I judging you for doing so? What do I really understand about your life and how you've come to this point. Why is it worse for you to use a prostitute than anyone else? Is this my business at all? I don't grill other patients about whom they are planning to use Viagra with. You're entitled to your four tablets a month and good luck to you.

How can these tracks merge and if they do, where do we end up? As things stand, the relational track struggles to keep pace with the other three rule-based tracks and, as a result, can be overlooked and forgotten.

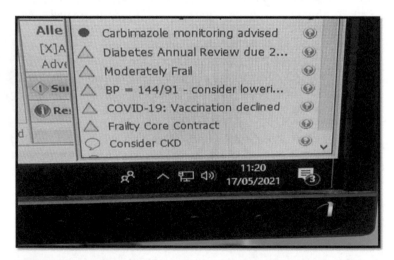

FIGURE I.3: The electronic patient record is not silent in surveillance medicine. It reminds the healthcare worker of tasks that need to be carried out and increases decision density. Rupal Shah, 2021.

Every day, we make hundreds of small, moral decisions about how we choose to interact with patients. Which track are we on? How much do we think about this?

It is impossible to step outside the system. But it is a well-known phenomenon that in highly regulated environments, workers bend the rules to get their jobs done. There are choices about how to approach the multiple, small daily decisions we make and the interactions we have, even if these choices are heavily influenced by the contextual factors described above. Are we healers or administrators? Advocates for patients or disciplinarians enforcing rationing? Scientists or therapists? Realistically, GPs oscillate between these roles throughout their working days.

The theme of this book – relationship-based care in an age of commodified healthcare – was debated in the House of Commons in 2022 (The Future of General Practice). However, lived experience is not taken into account in policy documents or mission statements, where politics has a capital P. We have used anecdotes in this book because they allow us to explore tensions and paradoxes using our own lived work experience. Our stories incorporate politics with a small p – the practicalities, logistics, and interactions GPs have with the artefacts of bureaucracy, which are physical (forms, filing cabinets, paper reports), digital (online templates, algorithms, etc.), and cultural (regulation, control).[23] In our line of work, emotional labour is never decontextualized – it is intertwined with administrative actions, writing, using templates, and making organizational choices. These choices have moral and ethical dimensions, which is why the influence of bureaucratic structures on client interaction is especially pertinent.

The Opt-Out Clause

Many of the changes that have come in over the last couple of decades have gone some way towards regulating care and standardizing approaches to prevent maverick and unethical practices. Guidelines and incentivization of chronic disease management have probably helped to improve population health measures and effective, safe prescribing.

However, an unintended consequence of establishing boundaries is to encourage a generic approach in which clinicians are reluctant to take emotional risks and therefore do not deviate from guidelines and protocols, even when they should. 'Work to rule' is what protects you when something goes wrong, but affection and accolades are given to the one who walks the extra mile. Paradoxically, walking this extra mile for the sake of either good care or satisfaction in work may necessitate breaking the very rules that are in place to protect patients and healthcare professionals. There is a real tension between the desire to provide individualized care and the reluctance to break rules, which results in the 'patient-centred' care to which we all subscribe being far from the lived experience of many of our patients. The irony is that our structures of governance fail to challenge or even to detect clinicians who follow the letter of the law; but who are not interested in connection and who don't give anything of themselves during interactions with patients. It isn't something that can be measured easily, unlike 'sort, fix, or send'. There is tension between the spirit of the law and the letter of the law. It matters. Street-level clinicians painfully negotiate between prioritizing patient-centredness (promoting the service user to poppet) or following rules (treating the service user as a parcel).

Students are exposed to protocol from the time they start their clinical placements and must make sense of how it fits with the diagnostic decision-making they are taught. The contradictory messages and inconsistency are confusing – 'manage uncertainty but do so in a way which maximises patient safety'; 'use yourself as part of the treatment but only in your contracted hours'; 'be aware of complexity while referring to the guidelines'. Jens explored the approaches of medical students in dealing with uncertainty in a series of qualitative interviews, as part of his M Ed dissertation.[24] What follows below is the transcript of a conversation between Jens and Louie, a medical student (not his real name) in 2019.

Transcript of a conversation between Jens and Louie

Louie: *In all of medicine there are now so many protocols that have to be followed, and I think they take away some of the clinical decision-making.*
Jens: *That's interesting. How do people deal with these protocols in hospital and primary care?*
Louie: *Well, my placement in A&E. You see a lot of patients that come in that the – you know the doctors feel that – if you speak to them, you feel that they're actually, you know, they're fine. They think they're fine. But the protocol dictates*

> *that they have a head CT or that they're admitted for a certain observation period.*
> **Jens:** *So the protocol is boss, not the doctor?*
> **Louie:** *Well, I think that protocol is – as you say, protocol is boss. I think even if a consultant doesn't agree with a decision – thinks something, if it contradicts the protocol, they would still follow the protocol because medicolegally, they're watching their backs in terms of if this came up in court could I defend not following the protocol? And most of the time, they would probably again rather err on the side of caution and follow the protocol, even if they thought it was a waste of time.*

The rules, guidelines, and boundaries within which we operate can ultimately provide an opt-out clause, allowing doctors to maintain a safe distance and excusing us from authentic engagement with patients. The computer really does say 'No'. We can use the boundaries to avoid taking on the burden of emotional risk taking. Realistically, all of us use this opt-out clause sometimes, but how often varies. A lot depends on the culture of the practice. There are always unwritten rules about what is and what isn't ok; how much importance is given to the rules; and how much we support each other. The everyday interactions that take place within a practice and between the practice and the outside world shape its culture and determine the implicit rules of how its practitioners should consult – including which of the trains of thought described in the case study above are privileged.[25] In a supportive team with strong relationships, risk taking is easier because there is more of ourselves to give. But even so, there are limits. We want to go home and see our families. We have our own deadlines and commitments. The lived work experience of GPs is situated in a system that has many rules, where protocol is King, and in which demand far outstrips supply. There is always a bit further we could go, a little bit more of ourselves we could give. In contrast to paper, digital platforms are not patient. They are active and demanding and there are consequences if the data monster is not fed in time (see Figure I.4).

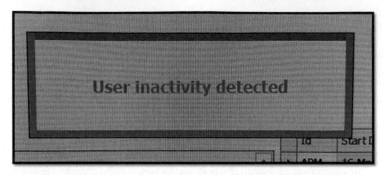

FIGURE I.4: Pop-up notice in the Adastra computer system – digital platforms can have disciplinarian functionality. Jens Foell, 2021.

In this book, we will illustrate through stories from personal experience, the realities of working as street-level bureaucrats, trying to maintain an elusive (or illusory) balance between following protocol, treating patients as individuals within a system geared towards 'Sort, Fix or Send'; and self-preservation.

Notes

1. J. Tudor Hart, 'A New Kind of Doctor', *Journal of the Royal Society of Medicine* 74, no. 12 (1981): 871–83, http://www.ncbi.nlm.nih.gov/pmc/articles/PMC1439454/.

2. Mary Winkler, 'Doctor and Doll', *AMA Journal of Ethics* 4, no. 2 (2002): 41–44.

3. John Berger and Jean Mohr, *A Fortunate Man*, 1st ed. (Edinburgh: Canongate, 1967).

4. Michael Lipsky, *Street-Level Bureaucracy: Dilemmas of the Individual in Public Service* (London: Russell Sage Foundation, 2010).

5. Stephen Harrison and Ruth McDonald, 'Science, Consumerism and Bureaucracy: New Legitimations of Medical Professionalism', *International Journal of Public Sector Management* 16 (2003): 110–21.

6. 'Bolitho v. City and Hackney Health Authority', ed. House of Lords (1997), https://publications.parliament.uk/pa/ld199798/ldjudgmt/jd971113/bolio1.htm, accessed April 4, 2023.

7. Joanne Reeve, 'Interpretive Medicine: Supporting Generalism in a Changing Primary Care World', *Occasional Paper (Royal College of General Practitioners)*, no. 88 (2010): 1.

8. Stephen Harrison, Michael Moran, and Bruce Wood, 'Policy Emergence and Policy Convergence: The Case of "Scientific-Bureaucratic Medicine" in the United States and United Kingdom', *The British Journal of Politics and International Relations* 4, no. 1 (2002): 1–24.

9. Jill Maben, Mary Adams, Riccardo Peccei, Trevor Murrells, and Glenn Robert, '"Poppets and Parcels": The Links Between Staff Experience of Work and Acutely Ill Older Peoples' Experience of Hospital Care', *International Journal of Older People Nursing* 7, no. 2 (2012): 83–94.

10. Simon Cocksedge, Rebecca Greenfield, G. Kelly Nugent, and Carolyn Chew-Graham, 'Holding Relationships in Primary Care: A Qualitative Exploration of Doctors' and Patients' Perceptions', *British Journal of General Practice* 61, no. 589 (2011): e484–e91.

11. Eric B. Larson and Xin Yao, 'Clinical Empathy as Emotional Labor in the Patient-Physician Relationship', *Jama* 293, no. 9 (2005): 1100–06.

12. Paul Crawford and Brian Brown, 'Fast Healthcare: Brief Communication, Traps and Opportunities', *Patient Education and Counseling* 82, no. 1 (2011): 3–10.

13. London Professional Support Unit, 'The Language of Connection', Health Education England, https://london.hee.nhs.uk/professional-development/specialist-clinical-communication-linguistic-services, accessed April 4, 2023.

14. Dariusz Galasiński, 'On Medical We', 2017, https://dariuszgalasinski.com/2017/12/16/we/, accessed April 4, 2023.

15. Joseph S. Collings, 'General Practice in England Today. A Reconnaissance', *Lancet* 255 (1950): 555–85.

16. Victoria Tzortziou Brown, Simon Gregory, and Denis Pereira Gray, 'The Power of Personal Care: The Value of the Patient–GP Consultation', *British Journal of General Practice* 70, no. 701 (2020): 596–97.

17. Daniel J. Martin, John P. Garske, and M. Katherine Davis, 'Relation of the Therapeutic Alliance with Outcome and Other Variables: A Meta-Analytic Review', *Journal of Consulting and Clinical Psychology* 68, no. 3 (2000): 438.

18. David Zigmond, 'Human Contact: Do We Need It in Medical Practice?', *British Journal of General Practice* 71, no. 710 (2021): 412–13, https://doi.org/10.3399/bjgp21X716933, https://bjgp.org/content/bjgp/71/710/412.full.pdf.

19. Rupal Shah, Robert Clarke, Sanjiv Ahluwalia, and John Launer, 'Finding Meaning in the Consultation: Introducing the Hermeneutic Window', *British Journal of General Practice* 70, no. 699 (2020): 502–03.

20. Havi Carel, 'The Philosophical Role of Illness', *Metaphilosophy* 45, no. 1 (2014): 20–40.

21. Haridimos Tsoukas, 'The Tyranny of Light: The Temptations and the Paradoxes of the Information Society', *Futures* 29, no. 9 (1997): 827–43.

22. Donald A. Schön, *The Reflective Practitioner: How Professionals Think in Action* (London: Routledge, 2017).

23. Craig Robertson, *The Filing Cabinet: A Vertical History of Information* (Minneapolis, MN: University of Minnesota Press, 2021).

24. Jens Foell, 'The Threshold that Connects and Separates, Becoming and Being a Doctor. How Do 5th and 6th Year Medical Students at Imperial College (London) Experience and Manage Uncertainty in Clinical Practice?' (London: Master of Education Imperial College London, 2020).

25. John Spicer, Sanjiv Ahluwalia, and Rupal Shah, 'Moral Flux in Primary Care: The Effect of Complexity', *Journal of Medical Ethics* 47, no. 2 (2021): 86–89.

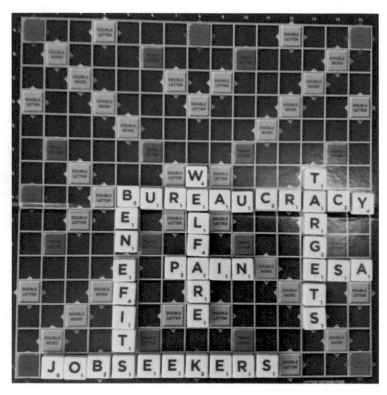

FIGURE 1.1: Scrabble 1, 'Bureaucracy', Rupal Shah and Jens Foell, 2021.

1.
Weaponized Bureaucracy: Bureaucracy as a Source of Injustice

Protocol Is a Weapon Which Can Be Wielded Against Patients in the Name of Care

General practice today is like a factory with a daily quota of outputs that must be generated. There are targets for vaccinations, for cervical smears, and for recording blood pressure, weight, smoking status, monitoring and treating chronic disease, drug monitoring, and prescription monitoring. The surveillance machine is working at full steam. These outputs generate multiple new workstreams: managing abnormal blood test results and abnormal smear results, recalling patients, answering queries about prescriptions, dealing with letters from hospitals with requests for more monitoring or referrals, a myriad of forms to fill in. The machinery is whirring, all employees are occupied, there is perpetual movement and noise, alarms going off, unexpected inspections.

In one section of the factory, the workers' remit is to solve problems, which come packaged as jigsaw puzzles, mounted up in piles which never get smaller. Each puzzle must be assembled and put on the conveyor belt fully formed, as quickly as possible. There is a standard time of ten minutes allowed for each. The problem is that the box does not indicate how many pieces the puzzle inside contains. The number can range from two pieces to 2000 and is usually somewhere in between. Often pieces are missing, and the assembled puzzle does not match the picture on the box. The conveyor belt keeps moving. What to do about the puzzles that are impossible to solve in the time given?

The workers can either place them onto a pile of rejected goods and send them back to the head office; or jam the pieces together, even if they don't fit, and put them back on the conveyor belt half-solved; or can lift them off and try to fix them in their spare time.

A fundamental but undocumented component of GP is the holding work for the impossible puzzles – the patients whose problems can't be solved in the usual ways, the ones for whom there isn't a simple answer. It is the families who live in chaos with internal and external violence surrounding them, the ones who have had mental health problems all their lives, and the ones who can't express their pain and frustration. The holding work is needed at the turbulent junction where the medical, psychological, and social intersect. It relies on constancy, emotional availability, and advocacy, which is informed not only by medical knowledge but also by personal knowledge of the patient, their family, and social context. The advocacy might take the form of seeing a patient regularly for a period of time, liaising with other professionals who are part of the official structures surrounding the patient, writing a detailed report or smoothing referral pathways. This work is discretionary since it isn't counted and is unaccounted for.

Returning to the analogy of the factory, the impossible puzzles are the patients whose problems can't be solved with the standard blend of investigations, medicines, and referrals and who are bounced back from whichever hospital department they are sent to. Of these, the poppets are the ones we hold onto, go the extra mile for, spend the extra time on – and take the emotional risks for. The parcels are the others and occupy the default position.[1] Protocol is a weapon which can be wielded against the parcels in the name of care – on a system level and an individual level. In a world where our resources for being open, vulnerable, and connected are squeezed out, the ways we protect ourselves as clinicians are visible and invisible. The stories that follow feature poppets and parcels and of most relevance, parcels who have become poppets.

A Disordered Personality

'I won't go and see a therapist again. Last time, when I looked up, I saw him staring at his watch. I don't need to pay someone to bore them.' This sums up Ophelia's experience with health services. She has had mental health problems all her adult life, was diagnosed early on with a personality disorder, and suffers from low mood, anxiety, and intermittent misuse of alcohol and cannabis. In her twenties, she had a few attempts at suicide, either by cutting her wrists or by overdosing on her antidepressants. A couple of staff members remember her as a teenager and know it started to go wrong then, but no one is sure why. None of us doctors and nurses who try to treat her understand what happened to her to start her on this downward spiral. At this low point in our relations, we can no longer ask, 'Hey, Ophelia, how did you come to be so damaged? What happened?' I can imagine the artillery fire of expletives she would respond with and actually, I don't blame her.

As a practice, centre stage in our interactions with Ophelia is the ongoing battle we have with her about various prescription drugs, particularly sleeping tablets and painkillers. She needs more and more of these and tells us she has lost her last prescription or that it was stolen – again. We all suspect that she lies, often. There is an alert on her notes warning any clinician who doesn't know her to be cautious about prescribing these contraband medicines – 'Benzodiazepine and opiate misuse' flashes up whenever her records appear on the screen. The subtitle is 'this woman is a problem. Keep your guard up'. The warning prefaces any encounter with her so that a new conversation starts with a boundary of pre-judgement and medical defences up before she says her first word. Perhaps I will change the warning to 'Emotionally vulnerable, treat her with care and caution'.

Although her tests and scans are normal, she is in chronic pain – in her back, knees, and neck. The pain stops her from sleeping and she feels that none of us wants to help her. She has a point. I struggle to believe her stories of lost tablets, and it makes me doubt the rest of what she says too.

The bottom line is that I don't believe Ophelia. I think she may be selling the drugs we prescribe for her, though I have no evidence that this is so. An uncomfortable thought is that apart from not trusting her, I don't like her either. So, I use bureaucracy as a weapon against her. I stick closely to the guidelines and protocols which justify my decision to withhold what she wants – 'the computer says no …'. I can't admit that I don't like Ophelia; that isn't allowed, and I am definitely not going to write it down as one of the compulsory case studies I have to submit for my mandatory annual appraisal. I am not allowed to dislike patients or if I do, it mustn't influence how I treat them. And officially, I am doing nothing wrong. I haven't prescribed inappropriately. And I have made all the correct referrals, showing that I ask for help when I need it and that I understand my limitations. I just haven't tapped very deeply into my compassion stores.

Ophelia has actually had many referrals from different GPs – to psychiatrists, to the pain clinic, for physiotherapy, several times over. But however much I refer her to other services, she comes back to me like a boomerang. Referring her is a way to stop her from being my problem – temporarily anyway. 'Well I've referred you, let's see what the specialist says' is a great holding manoeuvre. I can press pause now. Until she is 'seen' we are in a state of waiting, which is a substitute for treatment. Except that what the specialist says doesn't help either and we are back to the starting point, ready to start down another expensive blind alley. Healthcare services are not a good fit for Ophelia. Her pain is real but not in the way pain can exist in an evidence-based world. It won't be fixed by drugs and can't be proved. Her contacts with doctors make her feel worse not better, an invisible sprinkling of judgement landing on her shoulders with each encounter, weighing her down. Invariably, the verdict is 'guilty' and the sentence further disenfranchises her.

Most GPs will have one or two Ophelias on their books. They are the ones whom we dread seeing on our appointment lists. Their names are recognized by all the staff in the practice and become a byword for a particular blend of emotion, part frustration, part irritation, part discomfort. Encounters rarely end well – or they might for a period of time, but eventually there will be a falling out. It sometimes feels that Ophelia is constantly testing whichever doctor it is whom she is currently consulting to see when they will reveal their true colours and betray her, as is always the case in the end.

Some of it is a battle for the upper hand I think, of doctors and nurses wanting to feel in control – Ophelia's life has always been somewhat out of control and most dealings with her don't follow the usual predictable patterns. It is easy to call Ophelia manipulative and to use this to excuse us from having to engage with her. If she is manipulative, what does that mean? Maybe like us, she is also playing the game of health, with the aim of moving into the 'deserving' category.

Our position with the Ophelias that we come across is one of combat. We feel attacked – our competence, motivations, and knowledge are all held up to scrutiny by her – and we hit back, more successfully because ultimately, we hold the power in this game and it is one that she can never win. No regulatory body would rule in her favour if she tried to complain – she has a personality disorder after all. I wonder how many of the decisions I make are in the interests of clinical expediency (it really is not safe or advisable to prescribe sleeping tablets) and how many are made because I am feeling attacked or because I am angry or frustrated with her. It is a very uncomfortable form of introspection, and I would rather avoid looking into this particular mirror.

I am not sure how much her diagnosis helps her. A label-like personality disorder pigeon-holes people and the associated categorization of character and behavioural traits becomes self-fulfilling. I am sure the diagnosis influences the way she is treated by medical staff, to whom personality disorder can seem synonymous with trouble, short hand for 'difficult and manipulative'. She produces strong emotions in most people she meets. It is easier to connect these emotions to her condition, making it her fault than to remain open to the possibility that change might be possible and that maybe she doesn't behave like this all the time. If it's not her fault, then perhaps we need to consider the uncomfortable idea that actually the blame lies somewhere in the space between us. If her pain is going to get better then it will happen in a context which allows her to be someone other than the woman with the personality disorder.

Life Is Xerox
Moving from Parcel to Poppet Status, Deservedness, and Entitlement

Whether overtly enshrined in access protocols or score cut-offs (for referrals, benefits, etc.), the flow of patients or their stories through the system is characterized by turbulences, barriers, roadblocks, and unforeseen circumstances. And very few people know the

details of individual 'journeys', also known as care trajectories.
National Health Service (NHS) institutions are obliged to seek
feedback, but very little happens with this feedback.

Each individual healthcare professional will make conscious
or unconscious decisions about the extent to which they attach
or detach from the person they must deal with. 'Poppets' are the
favoured ones, and 'parcels' are the rejected ones. This is mapped
overtly or implicitly against the big service agenda of the NHS:
the razor's edge of deservedness and entitlement. Healthcare
professionals are paid by their organization, the organization
receives finances from the Department of Health. The Department
of Health receives funding from tax revenues. Taken back to the
two individuals involved in an exchange about giving and receiving
healthcare, this means that a complicated set of questions informs
the actual or perceived level of deservedness and entitlement.

Pain, disability, and access to support are a battleground for
these conflicts. There are a number of stereotypical situations.
Here is one.

Sunday afternoon in GP Out of Hours. A distressed caller,
new to the area, not registered with a GP, states she can't take it
anymore, something needs to happen, she is IN AGONY. In agony
(meaning the last stages of life, extreme pain, and suffering). She
states there is no transport to allow her to come to the urgent
care centre, and she is already taking high doses of all sorts of
painkillers. She told the initial call handler that she has suffered
from low back pain since giving birth, she also has widespread pain
including hip pain and neck pain, and she cannot move. Eventually,
after much fighting, she is categorized as needing a home visit.

On arrival, the set-up could have been constructed by the set
designer for a television drama set in modern deprived Britain, or a
reality show featuring people on the breadline, like *Benefit Street*.
There is the big dog in the front garden. The minibikes strewn
across the lawn. And inside, the assemblage of stereotypes carries
on. The peeling wallpaper. The meaningful quotes on walls, but
also tattooed on the skin of the woman in agony. She sits on the
couch, surrounded by her daughters. She cannot or does not move.
Her long, bleached, and straightened hair is pulled backwards in a
ponytail. She wears big bangles as earrings. She is very big.

Life is xerox. You are just a copy. So am I – I am also a copy. My
copy says, 'You see, you need to lose weight and take ownership.

This is your own doing. Now I will say something about wellbeing and enablement'. She is clearly a parcel, not a poppet. I will NOT mobilize emotional engagement and will NOT go the extra mile, or deliver the extra smile. She does not deserve it. She is not entitled. I will ping her through the system. I need to get on with my day. I am running late.

Well.

What will such behaviour generate if I unleash my feelings and enact my attitude towards her as a parcel? So, I must review my agenda. I acknowledge that this is an encounter between a middle-class person (me) with his clichéd well-being agenda. Exercising ... eating healthily ... buying expensive wine for unhealthy habits and rewards; and a person who relies on benefits and has to repeatedly reinforce her need-state to maintain financial stability. Am I unwillingly the frontline street-level bureaucrat involved in regulating the poor? Yes, this is the case, even though I have not chosen to enact this role.

So, I have foreseen this 'mission impossible' and harvested some crutches from the minor injury unit before setting off. It was not easy. Crutches are not just given out. One must be signed off as being competent to be allowed to fit crutches for patients. This is a box to tick. Crutches are in fact a rare commodity. And it is a job for physiotherapists, NOT GPs. I must break the rules to deal with a typical complex common dilemma: acute unbearable knee pain in a woman with pre-existing pain, disability, and morbid obesity. But friendliness, acceptance, and validation of the pain experience are what the new National Pain Guidelines stipulate.[2] They ask me not to prescribe drugs (she should be weaned off her drugs), I should BE the drug. This is not possible without me drawing heavily on my acting skills. This is what I am doing. I remember the actor I worked with when teaching medical students communication skills. He replied, when asked by them how he plays unpleasant characters: 'I study them and find something I genuinely like'.

I am using this technique now. And it works. I ask about the tattoos, about the daughters, and about her life. I have mobilized my curiosity. Using acting techniques and imagination, I can reconstruct how stuck she is and why she calls on a Sunday.

The irrational lack of deservedness has become something that can be dealt with. In the end, she did not even want more painkillers from me. I could interact with her predicament, taking it at face value. It needed imagination, not sticking to the rules. By breaking a rule, I could deliver the very service that rules are supposed to ensure.

Reducing health inequalities is what every organization writes on their mission statements. And I buy into this, donate to food banks, and so forth. What I have just experienced though is a modern-day take on poverty medicine, and my initial gut reaction was the reaction of a Victorian gut which thought 'these are the feckless poor'.

The Invisible Man

It isn't unusual any more in London to pass by someone who is homeless. If I walk past a man who is no longer young, who looks dishevelled and haunted, I am reminded of Jonah. Jonah is just one of many patients registered with us who have experienced homelessness. But as a GP, he was the first person I witnessed crossing the line that divides those of us within society from those who are invisible.

Jonah was 36 when I knew him; originally from Senegal, he had lived in the United Kingdom for more than fifteen years. His life started to unravel when he lost his job as a bus driver, and he found he couldn't keep up with the rent on his flat. His sickness benefit claims were turned down. This was in the days when a company called Atos had just taken over assessments for incapacity benefit, as it was called then. Jonah's assessor was not impressed by his history of knee pain, or by his depression. Neither letters from me nor from his psychiatrist seemed to make any difference, but then I wasn't familiar with the language I should have used and perhaps I didn't phrase my letters in the right way to attract additional points for him. The feedback I got was that anyone in his position would suffer from low mood, so in a modern-day Catch 22, being depressed didn't count.

I remember the uncomfortable blend of emotions I felt in my stomach when he walked into my room. A vortex of impotence, deep discomfort, pity, and futility. The writing was on the wall, and he couldn't be saved, certainly not by me.

Legal aid enabled him to get a solicitor, who tried to petition on his behalf – but again, to no avail. His life was imploding around him, and I was watching it unravel, helpless to do anything. At the time, neither he nor I really believed that he would actually be made homeless, but after a few months, it happened. I remember the shell-shocked look on his face when he came to see me afterwards, having travelled in from the temporary bed and breakfast where he had been put up. The glorious sunshine outside contrasted bitterly with the broken man in my room.

'But what shall I do?', he asked me, and I really didn't know. It felt like just standing by and watching someone drown in front of me. And he had nobody to act as his advocate, no family, and no close friends. It is shocking that things would probably have been different for someone else, who had more agency, who knew the right things to say, whose life was seen to be worth more. That was the last time I saw him – I hope this is because he registered somewhere else. His name disappeared from our list, and I never found out what happened to him.

The Man with the Hobnail Boots

When Keith was in the waiting room, he would pace up and down, infusing its bland tones with a sense of menace. Other patients would avoid eye contact with him, suddenly intent on looking at their phones or magazines. He didn't need to say anything, he just had an aura of trouble about him. Any perceived slight would lead to an explosion of rage and sometimes he would storm out unexpectedly. Physically too, he was off-putting, being covered in tattoos of strange designs and words I was never able to decipher. I picture him wearing hobnail boots and a ripped t-shirt but maybe this image is just a metaphor for my perception of him. He was the type of man whom people cross the road to avoid.

Every time he entered my room, I could feel my pulse quicken a little and a new tightness in my chest. It was difficult to make a judgement during a consultation about the level of threat that Keith posed. He came into my room angry, muttering obscenities under his breath, '****ing hell ****ing bastards. ****ing making my life hell'.

Would I need to involve the police this time? I surreptitiously checked that I could reach the alarm button if needed, positioning myself between him and the door.

'Hello Keith. What's going on?'

'Those ****ing c****. They are seriously taking the piss now. I just need a bit of ****ing peace and quiet. Is that too much to ask for ****'s sake? They play that ****ing music just to wind me up.

I think I'm going to go up there and ****ing turn the volume down for them tonight once and for all if you know what I mean.'

I looked at him, my heart sinking. At least I knew that Keith had never actually carried out any of his threats – or not so far anyway.

'I'm sorry to hear that, Keith. I know you just want some peace and quiet and I'm sorry you can't get it. You have had those neighbours for a while. What's changed?'

'Well it's not just them. The Council's on my back as well. And my benefits are probably going to get stopped. They just ****ing want to get rid of me, don't they?'

All institutions want to get rid of Keith. It wasn't the paranoia speaking, he was right.

As he was able to vent, his rage slowly dissipated, like air escaping from a deflating balloon. He even thanked me for trying to help him. There was some kind of trust between us, uneasy though it was.

There were alerts on his notes warning of violent outbursts. He wasn't allowed to book early morning or late evening appointments when the practice staffing levels are lower than they are within our usual hours. As partners, we had discussed on various occasions whether or not we should remove him from our patient list on the grounds of unreasonable behaviour, but had so far given him the benefit of the doubt because of his diagnosis – he had a cannabis-induced schizophrenia-like disorder which made him paranoid and left him with a fuzzy, distorted sense of reality. We tried to contain him by encouraging him to see only one of two GPs – myself and a colleague; both of us knew him well enough to understand what was normal behaviour for him and what wasn't.

I remember his battered, shattered face with the scar running across his cheek. Typically, he came because he felt that he might not be able to contain himself any more and that he would end up hurting himself or someone around him – when he was subsumed by his feelings of rage.

I used to imagine what it must be like to live next door to Keith, wondered how his neighbours managed it, and what effect Keith had on them. If I am honest, when I thought of this, it was with relief that I wasn't one of these neighbours and that I was protected from Keith's ragings in my house on the quiet street a couple of miles away.

He most often came in to talk about problems which were not directly related to his health. He was convinced that a neighbour's dog regularly urinated outside his flat and that this urine had seeped through into it, causing a bad smell he couldn't get rid of. He laid down poison outside his door to deal with the dog and then tried to rip up his own floorboards to fix the problem, but neither worked. The Council were trying to evict him and it was only his psychiatric diagnosis which stopped this from happening. He explained his problems to his mental health support worker but all he was offered was a voucher for the food bank, which he didn't want. Nor did he want medication to dampen the rage and make him a more manageable problem.

He lived his life feeling angry but he wasn't sure whom to direct his anger against. Mostly it was towards himself and he spent a lot of time reading the Bible, asking God for forgiveness for all the bad things he had done and continued to do. The idea of Keith reading the Bible surprised me. He told me once that he had been a terrible father to his children and had now lost all contact with his family. He had been beaten frequently by his own father during his childhood in Liverpool. I don't know whether his mother was around when he was growing up, I never asked and he never mentioned her. Writing about it makes me realize the gaping holes there are in what I know about him.

It was never an easy consultation, but it was usually possible to bring him back to some sort of equilibrium when he felt listened to. I am sure he spent most of his life antagonizing or frightening others and being excluded without really meaning to. Things didn't have to end up this way for him and I think that there was a possibility for redemption which health and social services didn't provide – nobody rescued him as a child and stopped the abuse. History repeats itself and abusers were often victims themselves once upon a time. Pictures of Keith's scarred face drift into my mind and I try to imagine how it must have been to grow up in the way he did, with violence a legitimate form of currency. The system isn't designed for someone like Keith. The conveyor belt moves on and he is discarded.

People like him end up getting discharged from every service he is referred to so that eventually the only mainstream institution left is the GP and sometimes all we can provide is a type of containment and constancy, for what it's worth. This is changing though. Triage systems like e-consult which require patients to fill in long forms about their medical history and symptoms before they are responded to – either by a text, phone call, or offered an in-person appointment – effectively shut the door on people like Keith, who cannot navigate them.

'Thank God that awful man doesn't come in anymore. What happened to him anyway?' An overheard conversation in reception today makes me realize that I haven't seen Keith for some time. When I check, I see he is no longer registered with us.

What happens to all the Keiths? Images drift into my mind. Keith is homeless, having finally been evicted; in prison; in hospital; dead ... or maybe he was reunited with his family after all?

My life as a GP in London is full of half-finished stories; populations in inner city London shift constantly, as people move into and out of the City. In an ever-changing kaleidoscope of movement, patients drift into and out of my life, connections are made and then lost, leaving me wondering how their stories evolved and what the denouement was – and whether what I said or did made a difference or not, whether Keith felt like a parcel or a poppet.

In Search of Succour

Zamir hands me a paper bag.

> *Doctor, your daughters will like this very much, believe me. You will be very popular with them. Accept it as a late Easter present, I didn't get the chance to see you last month. But please, before you give it to them, you have something.*

He smiles as he hands me the bag filled with sweets and chocolates. This has become a ritual now, the way we always start our consultations. I have given up resisting and instead smile back, pick out my favourite sweet, and offer him one too.

He is now in his mid 50s, his hair is greying, and the skin on the front of his neck resembles a week-old balloon, no longer moving in harmony with the muscles underneath. He apologizes for not bringing more, but he has so little. This always throws me off balance. I am no longer the lofty provider of care, but instead the recipient of such generosity from somebody who can't afford to give me what he does. I am humbled and glad to be.

He seems to wear the same shirt and trousers each time, which appear to be getting looser as he loses more weight – his appetite is bad. The practice nurse knows him well because she has seen him over many weeks to dress his leg ulcer and she is worried too. I can see a scar on his chest through the gap in his shirt buttons and when he walks, he limps. He has chronic pain from his past injuries, maybe heightened because he isn't sleeping well. And because his ex-wife doesn't let his son come to stay very often, his neighbours take drugs, and she doesn't think it is a safe environment. He told me once that he wished for some kindness in his life. Zamir is on an antidepressant for low mood. He has always declined counselling, telling me that it feels too difficult to express in English how he is feeling. The act of translation alters the meaning, he says.

He has many physical problems too but since COVID-19, he hasn't been seen by any specialist services. The letters I get back claim that different doctors have tried to phone him, but he doesn't answer. Maybe he is in bed, hiding from the demons in his head and from his drug-taking neighbours, maybe the credit on his phone has run out. Even if he did answer, telephone appointments would be pretty pointless. His English isn't good enough and he can't make himself understood. He is discharged back to me even though I have written to the hospital more than once saying he needs to be seen in person.

Zamir came to the United Kingdom as a refugee from Iraq. There are stories from that time which explain the scars, but I can only imagine the detail. His family were forced to escape when he was 20 years old, leaving behind their considerable material wealth along with the life which Zamir was dealt but never had the opportunity to play out. It is hard to imagine him being part of an affluent, middle-class family given how he lives now. He has told me how many of his friends and family went missing at that time, likely murdered, and he has described the different methods of torture which existed under Saddam's regime. He has explained to me how it feels to have had to move many times, always starting from the beginning again each time.

'I am a person who used to laugh a lot, but I have forgotten how to do that now.'

He feels that he hasn't been able to give his son the life he would have liked to, which causes an abiding sadness. The antidepressants are certainly not a panacea, but he thinks they have helped a bit to lift his energy levels. A prescription and some kindness are all I have to offer him. I am a witness to his story.

At the end of the consultation, I hand him the prescription and he thanks me but we both know that's not what the thanks are for – he knows that I am on his side and that I'm not going anywhere. The alert on his notes asking reception to allow him to leave messages for me and to squeeze him in when he asks to see me confirms that he is a poppet, not a parcel. Of all his dealings with various official institutions, general practice is probably the only place where this is true. It is a secret present I can give him, my response to the bag of sweets he gives me.

Keith, Zamir, and Jonah live at the fringes of society. If I were alone and saw Keith on the street, I would be one of those who cross over to avoid him. Even though I live close enough to the surgery to be able to walk to work, my world would never ordinarily intersect with theirs. I might not notice them at all or if I did, I would make assumptions about them based on how they look. The gap is briefly closed when I see them in the surgery and we occupy the same space, if only for ten minutes. But although they enter my consulting room, they don't enter my world. When my working day comes to a close, I walk home and they are gone, only resurfacing when I next pass a man begging on the pavement or hear about the government's new policy on refugees or listen to a story on the news about a man attacking his neighbour. If Keith, Zamir, and Jonah stayed with me all the time, the heaviness of their pain would be too much for me. I would end up breaking down, leaving General Practice altogether. But it's something I still struggle with – how is it that I am able to turn the switch off when I get home to my family and cast them aside? I wonder where their stories live inside me and imagine their ghosts resurfacing and engulfing me when I have retired from practice and my life is uncluttered enough to allow them in.

Tramadoholics Anonymous

Toni is well known to us. She works in the health sector and developed an addiction to codeine and tramadol, both 'sticky', addictive, painkillers. At one time, there were multiple requests, which resulted in restricted quantities being prescribed and multiple over-the-phone consultations.

She told me at one time that she was using tramadol to address her mood, and as a consequence, counselling and citalopram – a genuine antidepressant – entered the scene.

She lost her job because she stole codeine from her workplace. The last entry on the pop-up message on her electronic patient record warns me NOT to give her either codeine or tramadol. Then a query: allegedly, she has low back pain and needs tramadol. So, I ring her back. She says she is doing well, has been having counselling, and will resume working soon. And she needs tramadol for her pain. NOT for her mental distress – this was the semantic turn. It somehow puzzles me. I think, 'Do the hungry receptors know under what ideological social construct the molecule has entered the system?' But I am treating her and don't want to sever the relationship.

The conversation includes serious allegations and negotiation about her kosher entitlement to tramadol. My thought bubbles state, 'Are you joking, you manipulative pill-popper, I know you, always an excuse and moral contortions', and I am sure she can read my thought bubbles, even over the phone. Vibes always leak.

I invite her for a face-to-face appointment, with the intention of introducing non-pharmacological approaches. I am not hopeful that this will change the pattern of her consumption.

One day later the Advanced Nurse Practitioner (ANP) asked me to see Leslie. She had seen him for his neck-and-shoulder pain and had already prescribed tramadol before she sent him to me. Unlike me, the ANP has a good relationship with tramadol. Before upgrading to being an ANP, she worked for years on a gynaecology ward and saw tramadol at its best, with good effect on acute pain.

And Leslie had acute, unbearable neck pain. She also mentioned that he is an entrepreneur.

I have seen Leslie many times in the past for what is in my view mood problems, and behavioural issues. I am not judging by saying this. I am aware of his difficult relationship with his partner, who shares his bed and workplace, but has not accumulated wealth with him. And Leslie is bitter about it. In the conversation with me, he mentions this ongoing, accumulating distress. I identify and treat his sore neck muscles, myofascial pain syndrome, acupuncture hands-on. And NO TRAMADOL, amitriptyline instead.

It did not work. It did not last.

He reappeared in the query book, wanting his already prescribed tramadol back.

And then the ambulance crew called me, 'We are with Leslie'. My heart sank, ambulance crew! What now! Did I puncture his lungs with acupuncture?

No, he was still in distress. They wanted me to refer him to the pain clinic. To a musculoskeletal specialist. I said I AM the musculoskeletal specialist and I have already given him love, time, needling, and soft tissue massage but NOT tramadol.

I am informed that it is not only tramadol he wants but also diazepam (which is better known as Valium). Whilst I am aware of the practice of giving diazepam 'for muscle spasm', I am not convinced that it relieves the tightness of the tissues or the mood issues associated with the pain. And I am very much aware of the risk of addiction. In this instance, it was a conflict between my suggested way of coping with distress and his banking on the pills. I gave in and issued a short course of tramadol and low-dose diazepam. It is easy to prescribe and let people get on with it. But this is not true, because they might not get on with it.

I am a street-level bureaucrat, and also an advocate for the patients registered with me. This is clearly a conflict of interest.

The relationship I am describing is like Capoeira, half dance half fight, and both parties are doing all they can to manipulate and deceive each other.

Collusion and Collision

'I know who you are and I don't like you', yelled the angry male voice to me over the phone. It was one of those phone calls that trigger something. Throughout the call I had to suppress my rising anger. The Hulk was calling, and one Hulk only creates other Hulks. So, I switched to Samaritan mode and listened. And listened. Mr. Hulk, known to us as Jerry, wanted to know when his COVID-19 jab was due and claimed he needed it earlier because he has a mental health condition and he is on dia-ze-paan for this condition. And that this dia-ze-paan, which I personally refused to issue previously, has now made it to his staple medication diet on his list of repeat prescriptions! Its existence is now carved in stone; he is entitled to consume it without having to make a case to anybody.

Indeed, he has a mental health condition. Not just one. His medication list includes every drug with an effect on the mind and mood. And this is only what he gets from one of his drug suppliers, our NHS GP practice. There is also the substance misuse clinic, and there are also the unknown dealers of street drugs.

The caller did not like me, remembering a hard battle over the prescribing of diazepam and other drugs like it. Eventually, he won the battle by going to different doctors and he told me that his higher dose of diazepam has been enshrined forever on his list of repeat prescriptions (alongside opioid painkillers, gabapentin, and mood stabilizers).

But the molecules must have underperformed: his mood was erratic.

Like all practices we have 'zero tolerance' policies to protect staff from being abused. But in reality, we have almost endless tolerance. Jerry has been with the practice all his life, apart from the times he was in prison. His siblings are also registered with us. Something must have happened in the family after their matriarch died, says Beth, who has worked in this practice for 35 years.

During the telephone call, I could hear that he was sitting outside. It was not clear whether he was intoxicated. He shouted at children playing nearby. It was very tense. He definitely knew how to press my buttons and get under my skin. 'We are like heat missiles', says a friend who is diagnosed as having a disordered personality, 'we immediately know where the hot spots are'.

'He is a nasty piece of shit', says Beth. She looked after his mother and his siblings. She is familiar with every twist and turn in the soap opera of primary care. She has the contact details of his psychiatrist on her phone and calls her to corroborate stories or establish a shared approach.

During lockdown, Jerry got distressed. The illegal drug suppliers, county lines, dried up and the need to obtain psychoactive drugs from us, the NHS supplier, increased. Beth delivered benzodiazepines to him by hand, on her way home. He was distressed and very likely was withdrawing from the surplus amount he used to get from the street.

Should Beth be nominated to the BBC 'All in the Mind' awards for healthcare professionals who go the extra mile, who are simply THERE and stabilize people without making a noise about it? And only their eventual absence highlights the role they play in actively holding someone with high vulnerability and also high risk to others? Should she be praised for holding her protective hand over him?

Or should she be reported to the General Medical Council?

She is going above and beyond. Beyond what should be done, into the dangerous zones of litigation and sticking your neck out too far, so far that it could be chopped off.

Jerry did not want to talk to anybody other than Dr. Beth. In this phone call, I held my position and said that if he needs something here and now, he cannot pick and choose his preferred healthcare professional. And that I will look into things and get back to him. I did my homework and phoned him back and explained that the list of prioritization for eligibility for the COVID-19 vaccine is not a practice matter. It is decided centrally. When he heard this, he accepted the explanation. The vivid green colour of the angry Hulk changed to a more subdued tone.

Beth mentioned at one point that Jerry's dog is very ill. Is his escalating anger and irritability triggered by the imminent loss of an important loved one?

But matters progressed. In another telephone encounter, Jerry expressed personal death threats to members of staff. Whilst on the phone in his agitated and irritable mood, we could hear police entering his flat. He got moved to A&E, where he assaulted staff. Then he was moved to custody, where he assaulted staff.

We decided to go ahead with zero tolerance and filed for his removal from the practice list. He also got charged with threatening violence. It will be a court case. He will have to pick his medication up from a secure place twenty miles away.

He wrote a card to Dr. Beth and expressed his gratitude for the care she has provided over the last 35 years ....

She is retiring in the summer; she says after these years in service her emotional availability runs low.

The game of collusion and collision is over.

Kintsugi

'I am broken', says Greg. He is in his mid 40s but looks much younger. Babyface, comfortable leisure wear, snow white trainers. He lives in accommodation organized by a project that supports offenders on their way back into civil life. He asks for an increased dose of painkillers (he takes a potentially habit-forming medication called pregabalin) for his unbearable pain. The pain is all over, especially in his right arm. His dominant arm. The arm he needs for heavy manual labour in the construction industry. Two old fractures did not heal, leaving his forearm wobbly.

Kintsugi is a Japanese term. It is the art of glorifying what has been broken by fixing and connecting the fragments of broken pottery with a golden alloy. *Kintsugi* stands for a way of finding value in imperfections. It is a way of creating new meaning for objects that are broken and imperfect. For me, there are parallels with the work medical caregivers do with emotional scars and ruptures, with injuries, with what has happened in the past and cannot be fixed in the way of restoration, how things have been before or should be in the perfect state of 'being normal'.

I am collaborating with my colleagues to be part of a similar process for Greg, the broken man. Some people have found ways of being resilient (even though I dislike the word) in the face of being broken. They have found a way of working through the hurt.

In terms of treatment, he is somewhere in limbo, somewhere on the way to being seen by a specialist – who in one letter contemplated performing heroic salvage surgery as the next step. Having worked in Orthopaedics, I can read between the lines and anticipate a bad ending. A bad ending IF he gets there, and this is unlikely because his appointment will be postponed again and again and then when it finally materialises, he will fail to attend because he won't get the letter or because he will be having a bad day. He will then be discharged back to me. So, we have to navigate this in-between space of dealing with an impossible and unbearable situation. The unwritten superscript is 'Suck it up', but that is not on the cards. The last sentence in Joanna Bourke's book *The Story of Pain* states, 'learn to suffer better', but this is a difficult conversation to have.[3]

He is asking for more. Like Oliver Twist in the workhouse, 'Please, Sir, may I have some more?' Pain is a state of need, like hunger, like thirst.

I don't want to be the ungenerous and cruel punisher, refusing him what he desperately needs. He needs relief from his pain. Greg and I are in an intense exchange about the medication he needs for his pain. We are both uncomfortable.

Greg's statement of being broken has more than a literal meaning. There is more broken than the bones in his forearm.

Some bony tissues are not mending, and the same applies to deep-rooted emotional issues. We both know about his traumatic childhood, the drugs he used to numb his emotions, and about the five years in prison. About his life of crime and his life of despair. His life is still regulated by the penal system. His life is on hold. He is not a free citizen. He has regular contact with his probation worker, with the substance misuse service and with primary care; and on paper with Mental Health Services and Trauma and Orthopaedics. I represent primary care and invest in being dependable. I want to do better than what I have observed on many similar occasions, where addictive prescription drugs are mixed with other psychotropic drugs to escape emotional turmoil, despair, and suffering. We are haggling and negotiating whether to increase the pregabalin dose. It is a drug initially developed for epilepsy, and then used for inflamed nerves. It has considerable value in the prison black market. I don't think this drug will be right for the pain he is experiencing from the non-healing fracture. His bone tissues have not healed and neither have the issues he has faced all his life. Like Tantalus or Sisyphus in Greek myths, he is trapped in a loop of pain and suffering.

I would like him to rather be Freddie Mercury, to break free and to escape what keeps him locked in, to find a way out. New meaning. A new narrative.

But the escapes he uses and chooses are the escapes which are born from injecting drugs. The veins in his arms have disappeared. When the practice needs blood to check his liver or white cells, he takes the kit, disappears to the toilet and comes back with filled purple and yellow tubes. He has taken the blood from the big vein deep in his groin.

This is the problem in our conflict: at its best, I can be a legal supplier of numbing agents. At its worst I am his legal dealer, operating alongside the street dealers. I want to be different. I want to make a difference. So, I call the physiotherapists and try to organize a splint for his wobbly arm. This in itself is a majorly bureaucratic operation – but with two phone calls and a half-threatening, half-begging letter I can arrange a splint, despite the fact that he is officially discharged from physiotherapy and on the waiting list to be seen by the specialist. I write to the Pain Clinic, where the buck stops in the hierarchy of hospital specialisms dealing with pain. The reply letter states that the next appointment for him to be seen by a hospital-based pain specialist will be in two years' time. I respond to the reply stating that in that case, there is no need to offer him an appointment at all, it's like a promise to be found at the end of a mythical rainbow. But I knew this would happen, having worked in pain medicine. It is why I moved away from such an aloof and absurd system.

Many painkillers are addictive. Greg definitely has problems with addiction. It dominates his life, it ruins his life.

The agents of social control – probation worker, mental health worker, GP – try their best to scaffold his way into a relatively 'normal' civil life. (A colleague commented, 'what is *normal* – the setting on a washing machine?')

Greg and I have met on numerous occasions, sometimes like ebony and ivory living in perfect harmony, sometimes clashing. I have the mobile phone numbers of his probation worker and his mental health worker. One GP visit can generate at least 30 minutes of extra time trying to get hold of them and to keep them in the loop. This administrative overhead of 'continuity of care' is rarely factored into what it takes to ensure continuity, to ensure that this person does not need to tell the story of their hurt again and again and again.

He asked to be seen by a mental health specialist, but his case was dropped after the initial consultation – 'discharged back to GP care'. It reminds me of the status primary care has in most research studies used by the National Institute of Clinical Excellence (NICE). 'Usual care' or 'waiting list'. Greg is a name on a waiting list. He is waiting to be assessed by a specialist who might be able to fix his wobbly forearm. As his GP, I am his advocate, his pusher, his doctor, and his travel agent for his journey through a complicated system.

I phone his link workers again and hear that, after having given him many chances, his probation has been revoked and he is back in prison. I feel deflated, but not surprised. I had hoped to be part of the golden glue that holds the broken pieces together and allows them to stay broken but reassembled in the shape of a new narrative – of *Kintsugi* instead of restitution. It has not worked.

But unlike *Kintsugi*, the process of assembling shards and joining them together with golden glue is not a singular act of creating a new object. I see it more as a constant process of re-shaping, of a narrative shifting. Although it is the end of an episode with Greg, I hope it is not the end of the story.

'I Need a Report'

'I need a report stating exactly what's wrong with me' is Angela's curtain raiser. Consultations are mini-dramas and the opening statement introduces the plot. It is the beginning of my afternoon surgery and I have seen Angela plenty of times: in A&E, in the practice, outside the mental health unit, and often outside on the street, together with other marginalized people. But I have never had the opportunity for a thorough and meaningful encounter with her. I am aware of the encyclopaedic back story including various mental health diagnoses and encounters with all sorts of organizations of social control. The practice is one of them. I am one of the street-level bureaucrats working in these organizations. We all have obligations to the client/patient/service-user, to the general public and also to our organizations. I am aware of Angela's various interlinked conditions, ranging from obesity to high blood pressure which are partly caused by the antipsychotic medication she is prescribed. And the aching knees. And the poor sleep. And the precarious financial situation.

I could press 'summary record' and the printer would deliver a piece of paper with the main-coded disease diagnoses, including a recent alert warning us she has moderate frailty. But she is only 45! The code has been attached top-down to her summary record by an invisible hand, on the basis of her numerous unscheduled care encounters.

In an article about incapacity benefit reform, Claire Bambra, Professor of Public Health, writes:

> It is unclear how all this will play out, but it seems likely that the deserving/undeserving dichotomy may well reinforce and magnify the existing stigma attached to claims that are based on mental illness and may therefore further increase health inequalities. Either way, it will have important implications for the health professionals involved, as the validity of professional medical certification is being questioned by the government, **and healthcare workers will become increasingly involved in regulating the poor**.[4]

'Why do you need this report?'
'I need it for my PIP.'
If I give her the generic printout, it would be fairly meaningless. If I write a detailed factual report stating her situation, her

diagnostic labels, her impairments, her activity limitations, and her participation restrictions, it would take me about 45 minutes (of my own time, unpaid – whereas medicolegal reports by insurance companies are paid for by the companies) and there would be a high likelihood that it would contain inaccuracies.
I hear from disability benefit advisors that most reports by GPs are inadequate (to say the least). This is a problem: such reports may have a huge impact and may be influential in processes of social administration and clarify the medical situation of the claimant. However, if they are to be effective, the doctors writing them require a great deal of knowledge about the patient/claimant, about processes of social administration, the criteria and standards used in assessments of physical and social functioning, and the intricacies of welfare administration. Very few doctors have this knowledge. The point system of assessing claimants' functional status is not taught at medical schools or in postgraduate curricula. It does not even feature in psychiatry training.

One problem is that the process is geared towards an essentialist formulation – that is disease. That is to say, the forms require detail about medical conditions (how many; how they are treated; their effect on various functions of self-care, such as dressing, washing, etc.). Relational formulations (an analysis of her impairments in the context of her life history and life world) disappear in the assessment grid.

If people present with sleeplessness and low mood, I ask what they are thinking about when they can't sleep. If I am curious and interested, I may hear about the debt. Many people are too ashamed to volunteer information about their financial situation. Being poor has become a shameful state to be in.

'How much money would you need, if I were able to prescribe money instead of antidepressants and pain killers?'

'3000 pounds, I'm in arrears with my rent and may face eviction. And I am reaching out for the next food bank voucher.'

There are boxes to tick: 'Benefit changes', 'Benefit delays'.

This is serious and important. Every doctor would see it as an emergency if their credit card got swallowed up in the hole in the wall and their fridge was empty.

Financial stability and food security are at the foundation of Maslow's hierarchy of needs.[5] They are the priority, without which other, higher forms of well-being can't be achieved. GPs deal with these matters on a daily basis, particularly if they practise in poor areas. The Faculty of Public Health argues for better mental health for all and relates the mental health of the population to politics and policy: job insecurity leads to housing insecurity, which is a fundamental stressor and exacerbates mental health problems. As a GP, I am faced with physiological consequences, but my job does not end here. It is about addressing the causes of these 'idioms of distress'. And this must be about more than suggesting mindfulness.

In my personal practice, I have decided to give more attention to these reports as important influences in the processes of social administration. They highlight meaningful intersections between illness (what the patient feels), disease (the measurable examination and investigation findings), and sickness (societal response to health-related changes in social participation). If such a report is written properly in collaboration with the patient, it can be an important part of the therapeutic partnership. But it means 'going the extra mile' in an already overstretched working environment.

The space between work-to-rule and going the extra mile, producing the extra smile, and investing in a difficult but potentially rewarding relationship, is poorly defined. And the essence of the job is exactly in this discretionary space.

Every year there are awards for professionals in 'All in the Mind', the mental health programme on BBC Radio 4. We hear captivating and moving stories about people who express their gratitude to professionals who went the extra mile for them and often saved their lives – not by heroic acts in the emergency room, but by care and compassion and by being dependable.

I am going to invite Angela to come back to write this report together. 'No report about me without me.'

Reflection

Identity, the sense of being an individual person, is constructed by relationships and by one's position in society, a society which 'requires us to behave in particular ways and to be a certain type of person'.[6,7] Power differentials allow the healthcare system to play a part in perpetuating these stereotypes, by reinforcing notions of deservedness and entitlement. In 'Life Is Xerox', the central protagonist is typecast as feckless and hopeless, representing the undeserving poor. Unless there is a proactive effort made to recast her and allow her to assume a different role, she will remain a parcel.

Miranda Fricker first introduced the term 'epistemic injustice' to describe a form of systemic discrimination, in which particular groups are disadvantaged because their status as 'knowers' is denigrated.[8] Havi Carel went on to apply the concept specifically to patients, who are disadvantaged because clinicians choose which parts of the presented narrative should be taken seriously and what can be discarded.[9] Testimonial injustice is the term given to this form of epistemic injustice. Hermeneutic injustice is another type of epistemic injustice which arises when a patient's own interpretation of their symptoms is overlooked because they are unable to articulate their illness experience in a way which fits the medical world-view.

> The fact that I don't understand you isn't your fault, but mine; even your best efforts to make yourself understood are failing, not because of their inarticulacy, but because I am untrained in the appreciation of the sort of articulacy you are using.
> (Carel and Kidd 2014)[9]

When Keith says that his neighbours are making him ill, doctors disregard it or consider it evidence of his unstable mental health. There is no diagnosis to explain Ophelia's pain. Zamir has forgotten how to laugh. That can be cross-referenced against a mental checklist of symptoms of depression in the medical lexicon and discarded if it doesn't fit, or interpreted through a medical lens so that the meaning ends up being different from how it was intended. Information given in the form of anecdote is routinely reinterpreted. 'Modern healthcare practices privilege impersonal third person reports and empirical data over personal anecdote.'[9]

'Parcels', the Ophelias, Jerrys, and Keiths, are at particular risk of epistemic injustice. They refuse to get better and have been labelled already as difficult, manipulative, crazy, and frustrating. They are considered unreliable narrators of their own illnesses, and the pejorative term 'poor historian' is used to transfer the weight of misunderstanding to their shoulders. The roadblocks which they continually have to navigate can fuel anger and helplessness, which render their stories even less medically articulate. People diagnosed with emotionally unstable personality disorder feel that they are viewed by healthcare professionals as 'liars; attention-seeking; unreasonable/difficult; manipulative; a waste of time/hopeless; too hard to deal with and taking resources from other patients'.[10] It has been argued that being perceived in this way is the cruellest oppression of all because it 'robs you of your core existential self'.[11] These people have often been through traumatic experiences that are unimaginable to most of the clinicians trying to treat them – there is mounting evidence that being diagnosed with mental illness; in particular, borderline or emotionally unstable personality disorder is strongly linked to adverse childhood events.[12] These are very often the parcels that jam up the conveyor belt of healthcare.

In the introduction, we described the sympathetic professional detachment of the generic GP, working within a tightly regulated, output-driven bureaucratic culture.[13] But the disenfranchised and overlooked parcels need care – that is, the 'humane and palliative aspects of healthcare, [comprising] a wide range of responses to human vulnerability, frailty, pain, and suffering. [...] Its unifying essence [being] concern for and responsiveness to the needs and worth of the person receiving it'.[14] The inter-connectedness of practitioner and patient and the role of emotion in difficult, painful consultations should not be ignored or shut down.[15] It is ok to sometimes be moved to tears by somebody's story; re-engaging with our own humanity protects against burnout. It is also essential to be aware of how bureaucracy can be used as a weapon which leaves no trace of the harm it inflicts. Health*care* could be better achieved if the status of poppet and not parcel was the default position within the healthcare system.

Notes

1. Jill Maben, Mary Adams, Riccardo Peccei, Trevor Murrells, and Glenn Robert, '"Poppets and Parcels": The Links Between Staff Experience of Work and Acutely Ill Older Peoples' Experience of Hospital Care', *International Journal of Older People Nursing* 7, no. 2 (2012): 83–94.

2. Serena Carville, Margaret Constanti, Nick Kosky, Cathy Stannard, and Colin Wilkinson, 'Chronic Pain (Primary and Secondary) in Over 16s: Summary of NICE guidance', *BMJ* 373 (2021): n895.

3. Joanna Bourke, 'The Story of Pain: From Prayer to Painkillers' (New York: Springer, 2017).

4. Clare I. Bambra, 'Incapacity Benefit Reform and the Politics of Ill Health', *BMJ* 337 (2008): a1452.

5. Abraham Harold Maslow, 'A Dynamic Theory of Human Motivation' (1958).

6. Brian Brown, Paul Crawford, and Ronald Carter, *Evidence-Based Health Communication* (UK: McGraw-Hill Education, 2006); Sioban Nelson and Michael McGillion, 'Expertise or Performance? Questioning the Rhetoric of Contemporary Narrative Use in Nursing', *Journal of Advanced Nursing* 47, no. 6 (2004): 631–38.

7. Nelson and McGillion, 'Expertise or Performance? Questioning the Rhetoric of Contemporary Narrative Use in Nursing', *Journal of Advanced Nursing* 47, no. 6 (2004): 631–38.

8. Miranda Fricker, *Epistemic Injustice: Power and the Ethics of Knowing* (Oxford University Press, 2007).

9. Havi Carel and Ian James Kidd, 'Epistemic Injustice in Healthcare: A Philosophial Analysis', *Medicine, Health Care and Philosophy* 17, no. 4 (2014): 529–40.

10. Sheree A. Veysey, *Look at the Human Being in Front of You Who's Hurting: Clients with a Borderline Personality Disorder Diagnosis Describe Their Experiences of Discriminatory and Helpful Behaviour from Health Professionals* (2011).

11. Austin O'Carroll, 'The Triple F**k Syndrome: Medicine and the Systemic Oppression of People Born into Poverty', *British Journal of General Practice* 72, no. 716 (2022): 120–21, https://doi.org/10.3399/bjgp22X718661, https://bjgp.org/content/bjgp/72/716/120.full.pdf.

12. Carly Porter, Jasper Palmier-Claus, Alison Branitsky, Warren Mansell, Helen Warwick, and Filippo Varese, 'Childhood Adversity and Borderline Personality Disorder: A Meta-Analysis', *Acta Psychiatrica Scandinavica* 141, no. 1 (2020): 6–20.

13. Jodi Halpern, *From Detached Concern to Empathy: Humanizing Medical Practice* (Oxford: Oxford University Press, 2001).

14. R. H. Binstock and L. E. Cluff, 'Introduction', in *The Lost Art of Caring: A Challenge to Health Professionals, Families, Communities, and Society* (Baltimore, MD: Johns Hopkins University Press, 2001).

15. Elin Martinsen, 'Harm in the Absence of Care: Towards a Medical Ethics that Cares', *Nursing Ethics* 18, no. 2 (2011): 174–83.

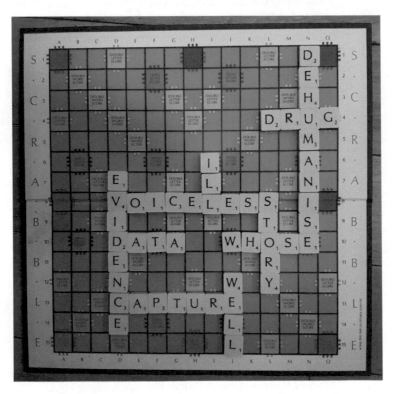

FIGURE 2.1: Scrabble 2, 'Voiceless', Rupal Shah and Jens Foell, 2021.

2.
Pigeonholes: Medical Categories

It is easier to talk about the diseases you don't have than about the stories you do.
> (Julian Tudor Hart, GP and campaigner for social justice)

The general practice of this post-millenial era is modelled increasingly on a 'Sort, Fix or Send' model.
> (David Zigmond)

The soul of the consultation can be obscured by protocol.
> (Rupal and Jens)

I responded to an 'e-consult', an online access request. The headliner was 'medication needed'. I did what I could NOT to give the patient what she wanted. She is in her 50s and works in health and social care. She looks after her father. He is frail and in his 80s and puts a lot of demands on her. In a novel, her situation could be described as a nervous breakdown. The day she requested an appointment, she burst into tears at work, left halfway through her working day and decided that something needed to be done. She was angry with her father and felt guilty for having these feelings. After a long telephone conversation, I invited her for a face-to-face consultation augmented sensory interaction. We talked for a long time about everything. I did not think she was depressed or that she had an 'anxiety disorder'. It did NOT fulfil my mental criteria of a 'clear diagnosis' as laid out in the guidelines. The emotional strain from her father, whom she loves, but who offloads his frustration on his nearest and dearest, his loving daughter, led to this. I was present during our conversation, no fobbing off, neither with tablets nor without. And yes, we talked about sleep, good food, riding it out, lovesickness, exhaustion, and nervous breakdowns. She had taken citalopram, an antidepressant, in the past. It's what she wanted now and it is what I gave to her. A six-month sticking plaster for not coping, for emotional overload. This is NOT what the guidelines recommend.

There is a well-established and substantial body of evidence directly linking chronic stress with mental and physical illness – from diabetes to hypertension.[1,2] The prefrontal cortex of the brain becomes stuck in a vicious cycle of constantly (mis)predicting the need to react as though to threat, without responding to the body's normal feedback mechanisms.[3] The stress hormone cortisol is persistently elevated, in turn leading to raised levels of proteins called proinflammatory cytokines. The subsequent inflammation results in physical manifestations such as fatigue, chronic pain, and low mood.

Lisa Feldman Barrett, a professor of psychology at Harvard and a leading researcher on emotion in the brain goes so far as to say, 'some illnesses that seem distinct are constructions: human-made [and therefore artificial] ways of carving up the same highly variable biological pie'.[4]

In the poem by John Godfrey Saxe, six blind men try to grasp the true nature of the elephant through their sense of touch, based on the part of its body they first come into contact with. Each conjures up different, but equally inaccurate impressions of the appearance of the animal. In the same way, clinicians usually see only part of the picture of someone they are trying to treat- typically focusing too much on the biomedical at the expense of biography.

There are many reasons for this, but in part it is because of the way doctors are trained to extract 'useful' pieces of information from the patient's story, which can be incorporated into a treatment plan. Every consultation model ultimately aims to distil and codify what the patient says. This is a stance which predates the rise of bureaucracy, but which in the age of Protocol has contributed to our current preoccupation with categorization. Havi Carel proposes that patients are particularly vulnerable to 'testimonial injustice' because clinicians choose which parts of their stories are credible and which aren't.[5] People who don't, or can't, fit in with accepted ways of expressing themselves can find themselves dismissed as being emotionally unstable or irrational. Clinicians have the power to choose what is elevated and what is subordinated.

Categorization feeds into how GPs are remunerated and this in turn renders it integral to the way in which primary healthcare functions. A considerable proportion of the income of GPs is now based on their work in managing selected chronic conditions – frailty, diabetes, chronic obstructive pulmonary disease, asthma, and hypertension for example. Interventions must be coded in order to attract payment and there are targets that must be achieved for many of these long-term conditions. The targets change every so often, and there are local variations. Many clinical software programmes are based on biomedical diagnoses rather than the symptoms which patients bring. Triage interfaces do similar work by pre-categorizing a problem into given templates. The system is geared towards diagnoses, and to managing these diagnoses efficiently and swiftly – sort, fix, send. This dominant drive to conceptualize healthcare as a production process makes it more difficult to mobilize the imagination to look for links and patterns or to see the bigger picture. The information infrastructure positions patients, receptionists, and clinicians in places where they are exposed to only part of the picture – the trunk of the elephant, the ear, or the legs. But the now disembodied elephant in the room remains elusive.

The story of the person behind the symptoms is not necessarily obvious. Maybe it was clearer in the days when GPs were more immersed in their communities and worked full time, with the whole family often being known to the same doctor. This local knowledge isn't as easy to come by anymore, now that GPs don't necessarily live where they work, work part-time, and are part of large teams – and the algorithm which grants access doesn't factor in continuity of care, even on an individual basis, let alone for families.

This is significant because clinicians wield invisible power. Judgements made in the form of diagnoses and subsequent referrals and treatment can have massive consequences for the individual.

Nora is a 52-year-old woman who complains of fatigue. The trunk of her story is that she has hot flushes and irregular periods. Menopause – give her HRT! The tail suggests that she is tired because she drinks too much alcohol. Alcohol problem-drinking – refer to alcohol services (coding this will have repercussions if she

> applies for insurance or wants to work in certain professions)! The
> body is that she has insomnia. Depression – advise counselling
> and an antidepressant (again repercussions for future insurance
> applications)! The ears are that she lost her husband to cancer last
> year. Bereavement reaction – bereavement counselling! And the
> whole picture is that her fatigue is a manifestation of physical and
> mental distress which is multifactorial in origin.

None of the individual categorizations adequately represent
the reality of Nora's situation and different clinicians treating each
problem in isolation might not work. The whole elephant will always
be elusive, even to Nora – but perhaps the role of healthcare here is
for one clinician with whom she has a trusted relationship to ask her
questions which help her to step back, make connections, look at the
bigger picture, and think about why she is feeling like this and what
might help to make life feel more coherent. Yes, there might be a
place for HRT or counselling, but Nora will have different versions of
herself and resources of her own which she might want to mobilize –
friends, family, hobbies, and ambition.

In his book *Beyond Depression*, Christopher Dowrick argues
that 'all human beings need a sense of meaning, of purpose, an
understanding of the ends of life, a belief in ourselves as valued
and valuable persons'.[6] In that case, the job of healthcare is as
much about asking questions which allow patients to explore a
better story about themselves as it is about formulating diagnoses.[7]

Being diagnosed with a chronic illness isn't neutral, although the
impact isn't the same for everyone. Potentially, the label of disease
can change how someone thinks of themselves so that they no longer
have the same trust in their body as before and develop a different
relationship with their social and physical world, wondering, 'is it still
safe for me to live in the way I used to?'[5] This is familiar ground – it's
very common to hear older relatives making comments like,
'I probably shouldn't try that in my condition'; or 'The doctor told me
not to do that'. There is a change from being in a state of perceived
health to taking on the persona of a patient. Susan Sontag wrote,

> Everyone who is born holds dual citizenship, in the kingdom of the
> well and in the kingdom of the sick. Although we all prefer to use
> the good passport, sooner or later each of us is obliged, at least for
> a spell, to identify ourselves as citizens of that other place.[8]

Life slowly becomes curtailed, as certain hobbies are dropped, holiday destinations change, and activity levels reduce. It is a slow, insidious process, but reinforced regularly by lots of reminders along the way – for example, the need for repeat prescriptions, requesting time off work to attend appointments, experiencing side effects of medicines, and declaring existing medical conditions on insurance forms. Havi Carel goes further when she says 'chronic or progressive illness is a comprehensive realignment of meaning, values, and ways of being that culminates in illness becoming one's complete form of existence'.[9]

It is not possible to quantify the consequences of this changed sense of self. There is an alteration in the meaning attached to the small, routine activities of daily life. You might stop running because you are worried that your arthritis will get worse if you carry on. A shared meal changes from being about social bonding and connection to an assault on blood sugar, internal organs, and arteries. Even the meaning attached to inanimate objects can change.[9] The pile of books in the bedroom becomes a chore to sort out or an obstacle that might trip you up rather than a repository of stories and learning. Nobody counts the effects of these small losses, which are on one hand relatively insignificant but which on the other hand all add up to create a sense of identity.

The stories that follow are about biography and biology, about the effect of medical categorization, and how we, Rupal and Jens, as street-level bureaucrats, navigate this discretionary space. This space has many voices and many influences, although the voice that governs uncertainty and risk is the loudest.

Ed and Lily

I became Ed and Lily's GP soon after I started at the practice, and they have been part of my life since then. Lily has been in a wheelchair for as long as I have known her, but she can still manage a few steps with help. Ed always leaves the wheelchair parked outside my room and they walk in, with her leaning heavily against him. He is a tall man, large-framed, and is able to support her.

Today, the pain which Lily lives with every day is clearly etched on her face, as she leans on Ed so that she can manage the few steps to the chair opposite my desk, wrapped up in many layers against the cold, but looking too hot now that she has been in the surgery, waiting to see me for the last twenty minutes.

'Alright, Roo, how are you and your lovely girls doing?'

'Not so bad Lily, how are you?'

She sighs, 'I'm a bit fed up with myself, Roo. My breathing's bad'.

The arthritis is spreading relentlessly, breaking down her joints, tiring her out. And now her heart is weakening, the result of a 'silent' heart attack some time ago.

Ed puts his hand on her shoulder.

'Don't be like that, Lils. It's not all doom and gloom. Roo's gonna think you're ready for the knackers' yard if you go on like that.' He looks directly at me. 'Roo, you're gonna sort Lily out aren't you, love? Do me a favour and tell her she doesn't have to worry so much, will you?' He smiles, hopefully.

I feel the responsibility of what Ed asks of me. I am invested in Ed and Lily; maybe more than I am with most other patients I see. Ed and Lily met when she was 13 and he was 14. She and her family had just moved to the area and she spotted him soon after this, delivering newspapers on his bike, the most handsome boy she had ever seen. She told him she was lost and asked him to help her get home – he called her a dozy cow but walked her back to her front door. It was the start of something. Ed had recently moved back to London after a long separation from his birth family when he was evacuated to Devon during the Second World War. Coming back home had been a strange and lonely experience. Meeting Lily was what he needed to anchor him and they were married within three years of their first meeting. Through the ups and downs, their marriage stayed solid. It is the type of relationship in which two people are so intertwined that it isn't clear where one starts and the other ends. Even in the tough times, Ed has told me that there was never a question that they wouldn't be together. They have four children, ten grandchildren, and a couple of great-grandchildren. All from that meeting of two teenagers who found each other more than 60 years ago.

But now her arthritis has taken a stealthy, insidious hold over her body, affecting her knees, hips, hands, and shoulders, wearing her down with pain. Surgery could bring her relief, but she is terrified by the idea and declines a hip or knee replacement. She is frightened that she won't wake up from a general anaesthetic.

The old, faded photos they bring in contain flashbacks of memory. Lily standing by the Great Wall of China, looking exultant. Lily being given a prize for her poetry. The black and white picture of Lily with a group of friends on a mountain hike in the Alps, cigarette in hand, arms around one another's shoulders. Her retirement party from the catering company where she worked for several decades. I have found it difficult to reconcile all these different Lilys. The young girl flirting with her new boyfriend; the adult woman who became a mother and worked in catering; the poet who loves mountains; and the old lady with swollen limbs and wrinkled skin who is bound to her wheelchair.

When I first met Ed and Lily, reality seemed to me to be fixed in the present. When I looked at Lily, I couldn't imagine the earlier versions of her; instead, I only saw an elderly woman whose heart no longer beat as strongly as it should and whose body had let her down. But as I have got to know her and hear her life stories over multiple appointments, there has been a shift so that I'm not so anchored in the present anymore. I am more inclined to ask what matters to her rather than what the matter is. And the answer is that she knows her body is slowly giving up and that her time is limited. She wants to spend every moment she has left with her family. She would rather live with her joint pain and breathlessness than have any intervention that is going to mean spending time in hospital. When you don't have very much of it, like money, time should be spent carefully.

So, Lily doesn't want hospital appointments if she can avoid them. She doesn't want me to refer her for investigations if at all possible. This has been becoming more of an issue as her health has declined slowly over the years I have known her. It is quite an ordeal for her to even get to hospital and I have to remind myself not to underestimate the inconvenience of a 'routine' appointment. Waiting for hours in an outpatient clinic literally ruins her day; and when time is limited, this matters, particularly if the appointment doesn't change much.

When things are bad, she finds that writing a poem can distract her from her pain. And she is the one that her extended family turns to for advice. She is still needed and it gives her life meaning.

All the staff at the practice adore Lily and she has got to know many of them well over the years. I remember many random acts of kindness, which she was responsible for and also which she was the recipient of. The reception staff miraculously find a way to fit her in for an appointment when it is convenient for her. Healthcare assistants remember that she finds it painful to have her blood pressure taken with an electronic machine and check it manually without needing to be reminded. Nurses apply dressings with special gentleness, taking care when handling her swollen limbs not to make her pain worse.

Most of what I can do for Lily is to be her advocate and travel agent through the parkour of health services, to help her avoid the hospital appointments she hates when this is reasonable, and to tell her when I think it isn't; to remind her that she still has a clear purpose to her life; to prescribe for her so that her pain and breathing are controlled; to remember how her medicines interact with one another and with her illnesses; hold onto the uncertainty of whether or not I am getting it right; and to do nothing when it feels like better medicine than doing something.

Filling the Void

We've been here before. We look at each other, combatants ready to take up arms, but hoping this time will be different.

I must have seen Rosemary Williams a hundred times or more over the years since I first joined the surgery. She has arthritis caused by her psoriasis, which has left her with pain in her hands and spine. She also has ulcerative colitis, an inflammatory condition of the bowels, which when it flares up can cause diarrhoea and bleeding from the rectum. The colitis increases her chances of developing bowel cancer.

She is a small, slight woman, always dressed in several layers to combat the cold even at the height of summer – she hasn't any extra padding to keep her warm. She is a bit hunched over and she walks slowly, with small, tentative steps.

She has seen me about once a month on average for years, always with new symptoms and questions about her physical health. She seems to exude anxiety each time about what might be wrong with her. Rosemary's anxiety often transfers to me when she describes sinister-sounding symptoms for which it is difficult to find an explanation. I worry I will miss something important. Because of her existing illnesses, she is at increased risk of complications ranging from heart disease to cancer. Most of her different symptoms could be caused by a serious disease. I know that she worries a lot about what might happen to her and how she would manage if she got worse. I am left after these consultations with a feeling of exasperation. Unreasonably, I feel as though it is me as well as her who is being attacked by her physical symptoms, which seem to multiply inexorably, like a swarm of midges buzzing around me. How can I fit her into a neat box and code a diagnosis on her computer records when she keeps jumping around from one set of symptoms to another? Why can't she make up her mind?

Over the years I have got to know quite a lot about her background, especially because once or twice, I have had to write insurance reports for her. Medical records are like an encyclopaedia of someone's health. They contain details of every illness that a patient has had since the time they first registered with a UK NHS GP. The old letters from specialists in hospitals which have often turned a pale sepia over time tell a story, sometimes unexpected, of every medical encounter over an entire lifetime. They can unfold like a novel, as you read about the childhood pains which turned into adulthood distress; about anxious or angry parents, rebellious siblings, and family strife. Mostly, GPs don't have time to read their patients' old notes – it's something which happens rarely unless a report is needed. This is a shame because doing so fills in background details of someone which might never otherwise come to light. Adverse childhood experiences like being subjected to violence or neglect can rewire the brain so that people become trapped in a cycle of constantly predicting threat, with the release of inflammatory chemicals that can cause chronic physical and mental health problems.

I already knew that Rosemary had spent her working life in various administrative jobs before taking early retirement in her 50s. I knew that she was divorced and had two grown-up sons who lived not too far away from her, in nearby suburbs of London; and that she was hoping for grandchildren to arrive soon, now that both boys were settled down with partners. Through reading her notes, I also found out that she had bad asthma as a child, which she eventually grew out of. She missed so much school that she left at the age of 15 without any qualifications. 'Unsurprisingly, Rosemary has now left school without succeeding in obtaining any O'levels', a respiratory consultant noted in a clinic letter. There was an addendum stating that Rosemary was now in foster care and was no longer in touch with her birth family.

This was at a time when the class divide between most doctors and their patients was even more pronounced than it is today. Doctors overtly wielded power, especially over people like Rosemary – and there was no need to temper their thoughts before translating them to a letter. When I was studying gynaecology as a medical student, there was a teenager who had been admitted for pelvic inflammatory disease caused by the chlamydia infection she had picked up from her boyfriend. My 'firm' of students saw her on our teaching ward round with the consultant and he asked us what was wrong with her. We offered different possible diagnoses. 'No, no', he smirked. 'What's wrong with her is that she's a loser.' She was two feet away from him and there is no possibility she didn't hear. He wouldn't get away with that now, although we haven't yet worked out a way to police thoughts.

Rosemary has had dozens of hospital referrals over the years, each accompanied by multiple investigations, which have fuelled her anxiety. Some were probably necessary, and some were not. Some were repetitious, some were done for no obvious reason. Referring her to a specialist means that there is a 'plan' in place so that we can both fool ourselves with the idea that her problems will miraculously be solved by the 'specialist' she sees in her next outpatient appointment. While she is waiting for an appointment and she comes in with a new pain, I can say to her, 'Well you're going to see the consultant (magician) soon. Maybe she'll have an answer for you'. Or maybe not.

I have taken Rosemary's anxiety at face value and have thought it is probably a natural response to her physical diseases. But there has always been a sense of something unfinished and incomplete after I've seen her. It is a vague sense I have that I am failing her, even though all the boxes have been ticked and the right investigations done. But I haven't spent much time trying to work out where this sense of failure comes from. I don't look forward to seeing her. I have never had a consultation with her which has taken less than twenty minutes and even so ... if I am honest, it doesn't feel like time well spent. I have known that there is something else, beyond all the physical problems that I've never understood. 'LISTEN TO ME' is her silent scream that I have managed to ignore.

I have talked to her several times in a superficial way about anxiety and offered her a referral to the local therapy service or medication, which she has never been keen on. But somehow it has never landed exactly as I would have liked it to. Possibly these tentative forays into her mood have come when I have been feeling overwhelmed and irritated by the number of symptoms she has and she has picked up on this.

Then today, the consultation turns out to be different from usual. Maybe it is the summer heat which slows me down and stops me from worrying that she might never stop talking if I don't interrupt. Or maybe it is just the right time. She comes in and tells me about her bowel symptoms. She has had a recent flare-up of her colitis and is experiencing some residual discomfort. I offer to bring forward her next appointment with the gastroenterology doctors. In the normal scheme of things, this might have been where we left it. This time, I take more notice when she shrugs her shoulders at my offer and says she doesn't really think it will help.

When I ask her what would help, she says 'you know, it would help if I had anyone in my life who cared enough to ask me how I am'. She pauses. 'I don't know if you know, Dr. Shah, but I was in foster care from the time I was about 10. I never knew my dad, and my mum [...]. Well let's just say she was usually too drunk to even remember to feed me let alone anything else. And then one day, she just left and didn't come back.' She tells me how a couple of years ago she traced her birth mother with whom she had lost touch after being taken into foster care as a child. She began to meet up with her every few weeks, hoping to establish a relationship and fill the void that she knew had always been there. Her mother though has the same relationship with alcohol now as she did when Rosemary was young. It soon became apparent where the money she borrowed from Rosemary was going. Rosemary knew her sons would be angry if they found out that she was giving her mother money – they had been opposed to her even tracing her mother and were not interested in starting up any kind of relationship with their grandmother. So she didn't tell them – or anybody else, because she was too ashamed and embarrassed.

She tells me she has spent her life waiting for some kind of explanation from her mother about why she had abandoned her and whether she had ever loved her. Talking about it to me, it dawns on her that this is why she still sees her mother, that she still holds out some hope that she will one day give her answers which will make everything else fall into place.

She looks at me and says, 'You come to a point in your life when you just really need to understand what everything has been for, what it has all meant. I feel like only she can tell me that. If your own mother can't love you, who can? It makes you feel pretty worthless really'. Her words echo through the room, filling the long silence which follows.

Eventually, we start talking again – about what life might be like if nothing changes, whether she will ever get her explanations from her mother, and whether the void she talked about could be filled in any other way. She leaves the room smiling and we hug briefly, which we have never done before. She thanks me before she goes and says I have really helped her.

Rosemary is a middle-aged woman who was abandoned by her mother but who has still been a good mother to her own two sons, who has had friendships in and out of work, whose marriage fell apart, who expects to be a grandmother, who has two long-term medical conditions, one of which make her bowels inflamed and irritated from time to time; and the other of which causes her to have intermittent problems with her skin and joints. Her childhood trauma has probably contributed to the physical problems she has. But I have been trained to make a diagnosis and to use that to classify people. Her ulcerative colitis and psoriasis are the only two things which give me disease categories to slot her into. Rosemary isn't contained within these slots though, however hard I try to force her into them.

Life is messy and illness is complex.

It can take a long time to make the connection between painful events in the past and current symptoms. It is easier to keep discovering what people don't have than to find out what is making them ill.

It can be gratifying as a doctor to treat emergencies, to fix something which is obviously broken – and then walk away as a hero. My role as a GP isn't always to fix medical problems though. Sometimes symptoms don't have a medical cause. Sometimes people want me to step away from my stethoscope and approach them in a different way. Walking alongside someone and bearing witness, listening to and asking about their story is an overlooked treatment option – valuing the interaction, not just the intervention.

I'm Tired All the Time

Carrie is the same age as me and we have progressed to middle age together. Her children are the same age as mine, I remember when they were babies, coming in with colds and earache. She must remember when I was pregnant, both of us experiencing backache and sleepless nights. She always asked how I was before telling me what was bothering her, and I appreciated that because it felt genuine.

I haven't seen her for several years and seeing her name on the appointment list takes me back in time. 'I wonder how she is', I think to myself. 'And how are those boys of hers?' It gives me a jolt to realize that her toddlers will now be teenagers. People slip out of your mind if you haven't seen them for some time.

When I go out to the waiting room to call her in, it's clear that she has aged. Her muscles are less taut, she has wrinkles under her eyes and she looks shorter than I remember. Instead of the mini skirt I recall, she is wearing tracksuit bottoms. Perhaps she thinks similar thoughts about me as we walk companionably to my room together, side by side. I wonder how I appear to her, who knew me in a different phase of my life. The smile we give each other acknowledges this shared history. Life has happened to us both and the days of nappies have yielded to other preoccupations. It turns out that she is now a single mother, trying to manage alone after her husband left – she tells me that happened three years ago. It was a surprise when he actually went – but maybe not when she thinks about it. I remember him too, a small man, who tended to interrupt her and talk over her.

She isn't depressed but feels worn out and wonders if there is anything wrong, maybe she is anaemic or has a thyroid disorder. 'You know how it is', she shrugs. 'I go to bed wiped out, practically fall asleep before my head hits the pillow. And then it feels like the alarm goes off about 5 minutes later. This doesn't feel like me. I just feel tired all the time. How did I get so old?' She laughs as she says this, and the years fall away.

I ask her about what else is happening in her life. 'I'm still working as a teaching assistant, I never did get my teaching qualification – I've just been too caught up with the boys, sorting stuff out with my ex and then ...', she pauses. 'My lovely dad passed away last year.' She looks down as this sadness hits her again.

She is a single mother now to three boys and their flat feels as though it is bursting at the seams. Everything falls to her, there is no one to take any of the burden away. She is under more pressure than she realizes, and it is making her tired. She doesn't miss her ex, but being alone means there is nobody to tell her to relax while they sort out dinner or help the boys with their homework or organize the food shopping for the week. She can manage all of it, but it would be nice not to have to all the time.

We talk, discuss her blood test results which are normal, and then I suggest that she considers making time for herself when she can, now that the boys are a bit older; maybe pick up the teaching qualification again. I think she would be a really good teacher and I tell her that. If she believes me, it is because I have known her for a long time. There are no more investigations needed, the tiredness does not fit into a medical category.

Our lives intersect and then come apart again. I wonder when I will next see her. It strikes me how different the consultation would have been today if we had never had the chance to get to know each other all those years ago; and I feel sorry that with continuity of care becoming less common and doctors being less likely to remain working in the same surgery permanently, GPs coming through their training now may not get a chance to see the long view that I have had.

It's Only Arthritis

Asif is 52 years old and he wears his bald patch with confidence. He exercises enough to have kept any middle-aged spread at bay. He is the director of a successful company, his second marriage is to a woman 13 years younger than him and they have two small boys. He doesn't like to be kept waiting, practically runs into my room, and I sit straighter and talk more quickly when he is with me.

Asif expects people to convince him about why he should take them seriously. It's like that when I am talking to him about his health. It is very important to Asif to take his sons to the park to play football at weekends; he doesn't want to be an older dad who doesn't have the energy. He runs every day and has entered three marathons in the past five years as well as a sprinkling of triathlons. He thrives on setting himself challenges – they keep him going.

The knee pain he has been having for the past few months is getting in his way. 'As you know, Doctor Shah, I like to keep pretty fit. I am convinced I must have just sprained a ligament when I was out running one time. Not sure exactly when but then I've always had a very high pain threshold.' I try to downplay his symptoms, telling him the pain is likely to resolve if he cuts back on running for a while and does some exercises to build up his quadriceps. 'With all due respect, Doctor Shah, I would like to know that there's nothing seriously wrong. I would hate to leave it too long and then make it worse for myself down the line.' My attempts to reassure have obviously missed the mark and I don't have the stamina to keep trying. He reveals his hand. 'I'm happy to pay for a scan, I know that X-rays aren't much good.'

The problem is that tests don't always provide reassurance. Asif is deflated when the diagnosis is osteoarthritis, the wear and tear/repair type of arthritis associated with ageing. There is moderate to severe degeneration showing up on the MRI scan but nothing that needs surgery, for now at least. 'But isn't that what old people get?', he remonstrates. In fact, osteoarthritis is not uncommon at his age, but he reacts badly. Having a disease of older age has aged him. From now on, when he feels a twinge walking upstairs or bending down to lift one of his children, he will remember that it is caused by his arthritis, instead of brushing it off as he used to do. He walks out of the room an older man than when he came in. The irony is that osteoarthritis is just a category we use based on X-ray and MRI images, but the term is laden with social meaning (in the same way as obesity or cancer). Actually, it is simply a generic description of a process which is inevitable beyond one's twenties. As with so many other medical terms, whether or not there is a 'disease' depends on the effect that the symptoms are having on the person.

Lessons from Geraldine

The last time I saw Geraldine, she was sitting in the resident's lounge of a local nursing home, wearing a stained brown shirt and baggy trousers, dentures out, and smears of food on her chin. She didn't know who I was and I struggled to recognize her.

'How nice to see you, Dr. Shah. I trust you're keeping well? I'm afraid I do have several items to discuss with you today, but I will try to be as brief as I can be.' That used to be a typical opening to one of our consultations.

Geraldine had always been a good talker. My appointments with her very often overran; she wasn't one to let anything get past her. Quite rightly, she invariably wanted to know in detail the implications of every investigation she had and would never agree to a prescription without a full understanding of all the benefits vs. harms. She was a no-nonsense type of a person. Her grey hair was cut into a tidy but unflattering bob; she wore no make-up and sported sensible navy brogues. If anyone else was put off by the hair sprouting from the mole on her chin, that was not her problem.

She had been a school teacher before she retired, and it made me smile to think about how this aspect of her character might have revealed itself when she was working. I am sure that any attempt to hand in a piece of late or sloppy homework would have been met with very short shrift. In fact, I often felt like an unpromising school child myself during our encounters, in which my deficiencies were held up to the spotlight of her uncompromising gaze. She reminded me of a strict teacher that I had at primary school who had always made me nervous and I was taken back to that uncomfortable time when she came to see me. She would peer at me over her glasses, take out a notebook from her handbag and begin, 'Well, Dr. Shah, there are several matters I want to discuss with you today'. My heart would sink. I was simply unable to argue with her, I couldn't even get a word in edgeways.

The decline in her memory was slow and subtle. It took me some time to notice that our consultations were becoming somewhat repetitive and taking even longer than they had before.

'Dr. Shah, you really must explain to me what these tablets are for.' She took out the packet of antibiotics from her capacious brown handbag and looked at me sternly. We had decided during her last visit that she should take a dose of the antibiotic every evening for three months to prevent the urine infections she was prone to.

'I told her that last time', I remember thinking. As is often the case with people who are high-functioning, she was able to disguise very effectively how much things were deteriorating.

I had visited her a couple of times at home, once after a fall and once for a bad chest infection. She lived alone with her cats in a sprawling first-floor flat in a converted Victorian house and there was a faint smell of urine emanating from the floral-patterned carpet. There were newspaper clippings everywhere; stacked in no logical order, perhaps reflecting the growing disarray of her own thoughts.

This flat had been her home for the past 40 years, ever since the death of her mother and the subsequent sale of the family house. The first time I went, I almost tripped over a mound of books inconsiderately piled up by the front door, almost as if they were intended to catch out unwelcome visitors – though she probably didn't have very many of these, welcome or otherwise. One of her foibles was her reluctance to throw anything away, so her flat was filled not only with her possessions but also with those of her deceased parents, which were now becoming trip hazards rather than poignant souvenirs of past times. She had lived and worked in our part of London all her life and had no intention of moving. After retirement, she devoted more time to local politics and also to the local history group, which she led with great enthusiasm. She was a crusader for social justice, personal accountability, and common sense.

Her remaining family consisted of a niece and nephew, one in the Home Counties, the other a couple of miles away in another London suburb. They saw their aunt reasonably often and hadn't forgotten that she had nursed her sister, their mother through a difficult final illness with her usual steadfastness. I don't know the intricacies of their relationship with her, but I imagine it wasn't always plain sailing. I suppose that if she told me off, she probably did the same to them.

She didn't want to discuss her memory with me and would always change the subject if I asked her about it, deftly re-directing the agenda with a comment like, 'well, it's perfectly natural that things slip away a little more than they used to, nothing at all to worry about. Now let's come back to the matter at hand'.

Her niece Fiona was getting increasingly concerned however and wanted me to take things further in order to establish a diagnosis and also to persuade Geraldine to consider moving to more suitable accommodation – she was getting muddled over household bills and dates, leading to various difficult situations in which Fiona had to intervene. This was becoming a real nuisance; the drive into London from Hampshire wasn't easy, especially since Fiona had a job and a family of her own to consider.

Fiona called me one Monday morning to report that things had taken a turn for the worse. Geraldine had called her, anguished, a few days earlier. Evidently, she had parted with a large sum of money to a con man who had promised to upgrade the heating system in her flat; she never heard from him again. This would never have happened before. Geraldine was abject with shame and humiliation and had finally been persuaded to address her memory difficulties.

Geraldine came to see me a couple of weeks later, a watered-down version of her usual self, downcast and deflated, her fighting spirit drained away.

She scored far less well on a standard memory test I performed during the appointment than I was expecting her to. I was sorry to see how the tables had turned for the former schoolmistress. Still, she was dismissive of the significance of the test result and said something I find hard to forget. 'I know my family mean well but they are making me worse. I wish everyone would leave me alone, I am perfectly happy as I am. [...] Ah well, that's not allowed so I suppose you better refer me, get it over and done with.' Not allowed. She was right. She had lost the battle – handed over control.

It was a difficult situation. Guidelines and local referral pathways are quite clear about how to proceed in the case of memory loss. There were potential benefits to Geraldine of establishing a diagnosis of dementia; this is what we are told as doctors so often that it feels maverick to question whether it is always true. I know that there are medications which can help to slow down the progression of some forms of dementia; that there are support services; and that knowing the prognosis can make it easier to plan for the future. Also, surely we should always be honest with our patients, regardless of whether they want to hear the truth. The pendulum has swung very far from the time when doctors would decide how much of the diagnosis to divulge, how much they thought a person could bear.

There were also dangers of not referring Geraldine. She insisted on continuing to drive, principally to visit an old colleague who had moved to the countryside and who, like her, was deteriorating. I wasn't sure whether she was safe to drive any longer and had advised her to inform the Driver and Vehicle Licensing Authority about her situation, which she declined to do. Being backed up by the memory clinic would make the decision clearer about whether to overrule her and tell them myself. In addition, like her niece, I was worried that it wasn't safe for Geraldine to live alone any longer – that she might leave the hob on or the electric fire. I imagined all the various ways in which she might hasten her own demise. Part of me was keen to be exculpated from blame by being seen to follow all the standard procedures and protocols. I didn't want her death to be my fault. I felt ungenerously that she was becoming a liability, to her family, to me, and to herself.

I was able to persuade Geraldine that some blood tests and a referral to a memory clinic would be in her best interests. She could no longer hold me to account as she had been able to in the past and gave up without too much argument. Even with this 'successful' result, I was left after that consultation with the sense that I had betrayed Geraldine.

Although referral made sense in many ways – both from the point of view of logic and of safety – I found it difficult to forget what she had said about her family (and by extrapolation, me) making her worse. I knew enough about her to understand that being told she had dementia would be potentially devastating, would derail her, and undermine her self-confidence, which might indeed make her worse. This feeling seemed wishy-washy though, compared to all the reasons I should refer her. A consultant I worked with as a junior hospital doctor gave me some advice which has stayed with me – he told me, 'before you make any clinical decision, consider how it would sound to a judge if you were taken to court'. I thought it unlikely that a judge would understand that I hadn't referred Geraldine because of a 'feeling', especially in the context of a car accident or accidental death at home.

I didn't have this discussion with Fiona, though in retrospect, I wish I had managed to pin down my vague misgivings and ask her, 'What effect will it have on Geraldine to know she has dementia? Are there any other alternatives we should consider?'

In the end, the die was cast. Geraldine was seen in our local memory clinic and diagnosed with Alzheimer's disease after extensive memory tests and a brain scan. Her decline from that point was rapid. Perhaps it would have been even without the diagnosis, I don't know. One way or another, she hadn't got around to having a conversation with Fiona about her wishes for the future before she started to lose her memory. They hadn't been able to talk with each other frankly about the unpleasant prospect of Geraldine not being able to manage to live at home anymore. Perhaps if she had, they might have been able to explore options, such as giving Fiona power-of-attorney, which would kick in if Geraldine lost capacity; a live-in carer; or adaptations to the flat which would have made it physically safer. Maybe before she started to lose her faculties, Geraldine would have been able to make Fiona understand that her dearest wish was to stay in her flat, even if this entailed a certain degree of risk and to ask for Fiona's help in realizing that.

Within six months of her diagnosis of Alzheimer's, Geraldine was moved to a nursing home after a hospital admission following another fall at home. It's not what she wanted, but she didn't have enough agency any longer to fight her corner. She was judged not to have the capacity to make such decisions. Capacity involves the individual being able to understand information relevant to the issue at hand, retaining that information, weighing it up and communicating their decision. Geraldine was thought not to be able to understand the consequences of staying in her own flat and was therefore placed in a nursing home for patients with dementia. Safety won out over risk, but at a cost. She lived out the remainder of her days in that home, no longer causing any trouble, but a shell of her former self. She would have been horrified if she could have predicted how she would end up and I am sorry that I didn't save her from it. I can see now that there were missed opportunities and questions I should have asked Geraldine, Fiona, and myself.

If Geraldine had stayed at home, she would perhaps have died sooner – maybe from a fall, or another type of accident. I think that she would have preferred it that way though, to be allowed to live as she wanted to until she couldn't anymore.

Reflection

Disease categorization is essentially a social construct which serves the purpose of managing care processes and gives symptoms social meaning. Our approach to categorization is grounded firmly within a particular period of time. Our understanding of asthma for example is very different now from what it was a hundred years ago and will be different again in another hundred years.[10] Homosexuality only disappeared from the International Classification of Diseases

(ICD) in 1992. There are many disease categorizations which exist now that didn't exist previously – ADHD, personality disorder, and chronic fatigue syndrome for example. And similarly, there are categorizations which have become obsolete because they are now understood differently and have different social meanings – neurasthenia, hysteria, consumption (tuberculosis).

There may be political and social reasons which justify the creation of disease categories and the pharmaceutical industry can exert influence. Fibromyalgia is a case in point.[11] Researchers did the job of standardization by formatting generalized aching into pain in all four body quadrants, alongside other bodily dysfunctions and devised a set of eighteen tender points.[12] These criteria have been revisited and changed since the disease was first categorized.[13] Fibromyalgia belongs to a group of conditions which describe and therefore validate otherwise unexplained disability, hence the link to the political and social. 'Long Covid' is the latest addition to this group.

There is a huge gap between the variety and nuance of human encounters with health and illness and the way these states are represented by disease categories.[14] The human experience has always been and continues to be interpreted through the stories we tell ourselves and each other. Medical labels influence these stories and the stories influence disease categorization. There are feedback and feed-forward mechanisms at play.

This is how Clare Penate, an author and a patient of mine (Rupal), describes her 'panic attacks':

I did nothing about them, until one morning on the train to work in Covent Garden, I found myself aching to barge through the other squashed, standing commuters and throw myself out of the open window just to stop a neighbour (on the same train) from her constant jabbering. The train finally arrived at Charing Cross station and I got off to find that the stone floor had turned into sponge. My feet couldn't pull themselves out of the floor that had morphed into quicksand.

How does one explain the feeling? It is like attempting to describe the pain of childbirth, and how when it has ceased, it is forgotten. It is an enveloping sensation that is utterly overwhelming and had me longing to crawl to Albert Bridge, to lie on the pavement in torrential rain, begging for someone or something to make the feeling disappear. It is a fizzing effervescence, as though a Coca-Cola bottle had been shaken and the top suddenly opened as the frothing liquid swirled and roamed around my body at a rapid speed from my head to my toes. The morning after the train incident, I felt as though I was on fire. My body burned and I convinced myself that I was going to explode with the heat and that blood was going to pour out of every orifice. It was an intensely physical sensation. Again I wanted to run to the river, not because I was suicidal, but because somehow I had to rid myself of the feeling and the heat, and I thought that the freezing Thames might help. My panic attacks do not make me think I am going to die, or faint, or that I have lost my mind, I feel sane but out of control with the adrenaline pumping and racing at what feels like a hundred miles an hour. I want to tear my hair out, knead a pillow, rip the stuffing out of myself, so that all I am left with is a quieted body and a rested soul.

'Anxiety' or 'panic attacks' are simulacra, which don't come close to capturing the lived experience. And if the nuance of the lived experience isn't understood, the therapeutic approach isn't individualized. The treatments which doctors prescribe, which are included in guidelines are based on an assumption that categorization reflects the truth. This is particularly problematic in mental health. For example, according to guidelines, antidepressants should be reserved for cases of 'true' depression or anxiety. It is more realistic to acknowledge that antidepressants are in fact often prescribed as tools for people who cannot cope, as agents to appease overwhelming emotions, including anger – they are used to manage the vicissitudes of life at the interface of life and medicine, probably in the absence of pastoral and spiritual care, which could give meaning to suffering. Medicine has stepped into this empty space, or kicked priests out of the space in the name of science.

Notes

1. Rupa Marya and Raj Patel, *Inflamed: Deep Medicine and the Anatomy of Injustice* (UK: Penguin, 2021).

2. Emily Mendenhall, *Rethinking Diabetes: Entanglements with Trauma, Poverty, and HIV* (New York: Cornell University Press, 2019).

3. Lisa Feldman Barrett, *How Emotions Are Made: The Secret Life of the Brain* (UK: Pan Macmillan, 2017).

4. Havi Carel and Ian James Kidd, 'Epistemic Injustice in Healthcare: A Philosophial Analysis', *Medicine, Health Care and Philosophy* 17, no. 4 (2014): 529–40.

5. Christopher Dowrick, *Beyond Depression: A New Approach to Understanding and Management* (Oxford: Oxford University Press, 2009).

6. John Launer, 'A Narrative Approach to Mental Health in General Practice', *BMJ* 318, no. 7176 (1999): 117–19.

7. Havi Carel, 'Can I Be Ill and Happy?', *Philosophia* 35, no. 2 (2007): 95–110.

8. Susan Sontag and Heywood Hale Broun, *Illness as Metaphor* (New York: Farrar, Straus, 1977).

9. Havi Carel, 'The Philosophical Role of Illness', *Metaphilosophy* 45, no. 1 (2014): 20–40.

10. John Launer, 'Against Diagnosis', *Postgraduate Medical Journal* 97, no. 1143 (2021): 67–68, https://doi.org/10.1136/postgrad-medj-2020-139298, https://pmj.bmj.com/content/postgrad-medj/97/1143/67.full.pdf.

11. Gerald N. Grob, 'The Rise of Fibromyalgia in 20th-Century America', *Perspectives in Biology and Medicine* 54, no. 4 (2011): 417–37.

12. Frederick Wolfe, Hugh A. Smythe, Muhammad B. Yunus, Robert M. Bennett, Claire Bombardier, Don L. Goldenberg, Peter Tugwell, et al., 'The American College of Rheumatology 1990 Criteria for the Classification of Fibromyalgia', *Arthritis & Rheumatism: Official Journal of the American College of Rheumatology* 33, no. 2 (1990): 160–72.

13. Frederick Wolfe and Brian Walitt, 'Culture, Science and the Changing Nature of Fibromyalgia', *Nature Reviews Rheumatology* 9, no. 12 (2013): 751–55.

14. Eric J. Cassell, *The Nature of Healing: The Modern Practice of Medicine* (Oxford: Oxford University Press, 2012).

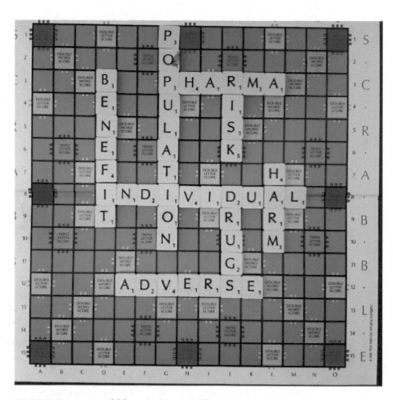

FIGURE 3.1: Scrabble 3, 'Adverse Effects', Rupal Shah and Jens Foell, 2021.

3.
Guidelines, Tramlines, Mindlines: Interpreting the Evidence

What patients seek is not scientific knowledge that doctors hide, but existential authenticity ... the angst of facing mortality has no remedy in probability.

(Paul Kalanithi[1])

The existence of moral ambiguity in decision making is not clearly described. The spirit of the guideline is nebulous, unlike its letter.

(Jens and Rupal, 2022)

'All effective treatments must be free', wrote Archie Cochrane in 1972 in the introduction to his influential book *Effectiveness and Efficiency*.[2] Cochrane was a socialist and epidemiologist. Ideologically deeply invested in making healthcare available for all, he argued for a robust process to ensure that only what works is universally available. He is seen by many as the father of evidence-based medicine. His legacy paved the path for NICE, which became a legal entity 27 years later. NICE is a non-departmental public body that aims to create consistent guidelines and to end the 'postcode lottery', whereby there is an unwarranted variation of care provision across the country. This asymmetry in the distribution of services is linked to poverty – the 'inverse care law'.[3] Services are often thin on the ground where they are most urgently needed, whilst the better-off may face the risks of over-diagnosis and over-investigation. After all, healthcare is a business. NICE was set up to change this, with the overall aim of improving health outcomes *across* the population.

This is as it should be. Healthcare is an investment in population health. Healthcare *should* increase the quality and quantity of life. But in a publicly funded system, what is freely available at the point of delivery must be carefully vetted. A lot is at stake when there is a central body regulating access to a huge market. Like a fast-food franchise where every burger looks the same and tastes the same all over the world, healthcare should be standardized with equitable access and fair distribution. The process of determining what goes on the menu of this health franchise needs to be robust and transparent. And each item on the menu should be both effective and cost-effective. The scarcity of resources dictates that only what works should be available free of charge at the point of service delivery. The organization's reputation is at stake.

NICE produces clinical guidelines, Public Health guidelines, technology appraisals, and guidance for interventional procedures. The targets that primary care services aim for (the Quality and Outcome Framework indicators, QOF) are shaped by NICE guidance. NICE also produces quality standards for medical care, as well as commissioning indicators. It rules over the process of standardization in healthcare and medicine and thereby controls access to the NHS market. It is therefore extremely concerned about the robustness of its decision-making processes in order to protect them from lobbying, undue influence, or even corruption.

Office and rule – both components of the word 'bureaucracy' – are exemplified and enshrined by NICE. There is nothing wrong with this. The organization serves the greater good of the population. It underwrites a utilitarian ideal. Jeremy Bentham's 'felicific calculus' converted a political ideal into a mathematical operation when he attempted to quantify the amount of pleasure which any given action could generate.[4] The felicific calculus states,

[i]ntense, long, certain, speedy, fruitful, pure – such marks in pleasures and in pains endure. Such pleasures seek if private be thy end: If it be public, wide let them extend. Such pains avoid, whichever be thy view: If pains *must* come, let them extend to few.

In a similar vein, NICE uses the quality-adjusted life year or 'QALY' as its currency to calculate the effectiveness and efficiency of interventions, based on the results of testing interventions in research trials.[5]

All these processes are based on representations of experiences – the processed items of information from trials represent experiences that have already been categorized, stories that have been converted to numbers, and lives that have already been rated in terms of 'quality'. Interactions between patients and clinicians are the raw and unfiltered material. Their representations used in research, policy development, and writing bills have gone through the process of categorization and have been organized in standardized templates.[6,7] Guidelines are deliberately produced on the high ground of research-informed theory, which may have little relevance for the dilemmas experienced in the 'swampy lowlands' of primary care, some of which we illustrate below.[8]

At each step of a transparent decision-making process, pieces of information get scrutinized for bias before they enter a complicated process of synthesis. NICE's workforce consists of information specialists, systematic reviewers, health economists, and wordsmiths. Suggestions for guidelines can come from various sources in the arena of health politics. If an application to produce a guideline is successful, the guideline is commissioned and follows a regulated process. This process includes an invitation for stakeholders to express their interests, hopes, and concerns. NICE appoints an advisory group, including experts by experience and experts by profession. Each expert must declare their personal, professional, reputational, and pecuniary interests. Transparency is key. Technical teams do most of the hard work. They vet the research, carry out systematic reviews, create evidence tables that illustrate the quality of information available, and set the scene for the interpretation of these research syntheses. The process of systematically reviewing the published literature, filtering the vast amount of information into accessible evidence review tables, and deliberating about its meaning for guideline production is extremely scripted, fair, transparent, and complicated. These interpretations then get converted into NICE-specific categories of decisions: 'offer', 'do not offer', or 'consider'. Another possible outcome is a recommendation for further research.

Towards the end of the guideline production process, the draft guideline gets sent out to the stakeholders for further consultation. After this consultation process, the finished product will be signed off and can start its life of influencing health and social care. Legally, guidelines should not replace clinical judgement in individual cases. Most of the time, they are based on population averages and cannot tell on an individual basis, who will or will not respond to therapy. This consideration is the task of the clinician who must negotiate between the lifeworld of the patient and the guideline. An important competence for GPs is to be able to critically appraise evidence. David Haslam, head of NICE, states,

> the mantra that I've given in every lecture is that they're guidelines and not tramlines. Doctors have a fundamental responsibility to use guidelines with their experience and with patients' individual needs to get the best possible overlap between patient-centred medicine and evidence-based medicine.[9]

However, once the space of uncertainty has been mapped and structured with rules, such rules can take on a life of their own.

To Refer or Not to Refer?

John Stevenson is an 84-year-old widower and a retired engineer. He lives alone now since his wife June passed away last year. When I picture him, he is wearing a patterned brown cardigan over a beige shirt and is stooped over as he shuffles in, leaning on his walking stick. There is a slightly defeated air about him as if he considers himself to be a refugee in the modern world, who can never get back home to a happier time. He has one daughter, who lives in Scotland with her family but he only sees her a couple of times a year because of the practicalities involved in making the journey.

Medically speaking, he is pretty well except for high blood pressure (BP) and chronic kidney disease, both of which are very common in people of his age. In fact, a couple of decades ago, he wouldn't have been considered to have high BP or kidney disease – the goalposts have moved in terms of our diagnostic criteria.

John Stevenson manages ok, even if his memory seems to have deteriorated since he lost his wife and maybe he is a bit low in mood. He avoids eye contact when he sees me; he keeps his answers short and to the point. It feels as if he would like to escape from my presence as soon as possible, in contrast with others, who have an air of permanence when they sit down. I wonder why this is. Is it me in particular that he wants to get away from? Or maybe his mood is worse than he is prepared to tell me.

I wonder whether he has always disliked hospitals and doctors in general and has preferred to let things take their course naturally. He has mentioned in passing to me before that he had some unpleasant experiences as a child with club foot, which left him wary of the medical profession. He does agree to come into the surgery twice a year though for a blood test for his kidneys, a BP check, and a medication review. This year, he has had more blood tests than usual, because a GP who doesn't know him very well decided to try to assess his general health, and give him an MOT if you like, even though he didn't have any particular symptoms.

The results of the blood tests are back and reveal an unexpected mild anaemia caused by iron deficiency. This type of anaemia has many potential causes, but one is a slow blood loss from an otherwise symptomless bowel cancer. A subsequent stool sample is borderline – there is a trace of blood, just a fraction over the normal upper limit. The national cancer guidelines suggest an urgent referral in cases like John's, to exclude cancer. As John's GP, I now have to decide what to do. John doesn't have altered bowel habit or visible blood in his stool, the most common presenting symptoms of bowel cancer. His weight is steady and he has no pain in his abdomen. He might have cancer, but it is more likely that his mild anaemia is the result of his chronic kidney disease or of a poor diet – he has been eating mainly microwave meals since June died and hasn't been bothering very much with fresh vegetables or fruit. But the only way to be really sure is to refer him for a colonoscopy, a procedure in which a long, flexible tube is passed into the rectum and moved around the colon to look for any signs of disease, including bowel cancer.

What is the best decision in this situation? The easiest thing is to refer him under the two-week cancer pathway, which is what the national guidelines suggest. For me, this means that I have followed the normal medical course of action (the letter of the law) and I won't be to blame if John does turn out to have cancer;

79

I will have done everything possible to expedite the diagnosis and will have nothing to justify or explain away when we discuss this month's new cancer diagnoses in our practice meeting.

Even if John isn't keen on being investigated, I am worried about what might happen if I don't refer and John's daughter subsequently disagrees with my decision. Potentially it might mean a drawn-out complaint, which will need to be defended and which will have a lasting emotional impact on me and my family. Receiving a complaint makes you question whether you should be a doctor at all, whether you are competent enough to do the job. It's really so much easier to make clinical decisions which reduce this possibility. I know that nobody will complain if I refer. The establishment will be on my side, even if John ends up being harmed – I would only be doing what I am meant to. And effectively, John has no agency to challenge me. Surfacing the moral ambiguity inherent in decisions like this can only happen if the spirit of the guideline is as clear as its letter. In fact, even the existence of moral ambiguity is not clearly described and so sinks into the opacity of NHS bureaucracy.

Referring John will result in him having further investigations, including a colonoscopy. To prepare for this, John will need to take strong laxatives to clear his bowels and to ingest only clear fluids the day before it is scheduled to take place. This isn't an easy or pleasant experience for an 84-year-old who lives alone. If a cancer is found, then John will have to make some difficult decisions about treatment. Does he want major surgery to remove it? Will he accept radiotherapy or chemotherapy? There will be numerous hospital trips and a lot of anxiety, whatever he decides. The amount of extra time all of this will buy him is unclear. It is hard to know how aggressively a cancer will behave when someone is in their 80s – and whether it will in the end be another illness such as pneumonia which will cause his death.

It isn't an easy situation to explain and it's an even harder decision to make. Having ten minutes to consider the advantages and disadvantages of referral – taking into account John's opinions and beliefs – and to convey this back to him is not really possible. To do it properly, and help him navigate the complex zone of decision making means several appointments and running late after this one. The anaemia which has been found by accident means that John's risk of having bowel cancer is higher than it would have been if he had a normal blood count, probably in the region of 10 per cent now, compared to about 1 per cent if he wasn't anaemic. But there is still a 90 per cent chance he doesn't have bowel cancer; and the potential harms of referring are not insignificant, especially since John dislikes and is frightened of hospitals and doesn't have family nearby to help him through the process; and that he might not want treatment, which anyway might not work.

Of course, all doctors would say that they want to do the best for their patients, to extend life and cure disease. But then, equally important is to do no harm. There are influences on my behaviour which are difficult to talk about – I want to avoid getting complaints and being criticized by my peers. I am thinking of our 'significant event' meetings in which we discuss new cancers and whether they could have been diagnosed earlier. It's not just me. Doctors are increasingly more likely to follow the more conventional, straightforward option of referring according to the letter of the guideline and detaching themselves from what the consequences might be. However, it could be argued that any decision that is made defensively – which is not in the patient's best interests but which is conceived primarily to protect the clinician – is negligent.

Preventative medicine – ordering investigations or prescribing treatment to detect or treat an illness which is not causing symptoms – is not straightforward. We don't know the future and we can't accurately predict the effects of the decisions we make. The GP who ordered the blood test in the first place couldn't have known that ticking an extra box on the form might lead to an old man's life being changed – whether for the better or worse is not clear. In primary care, an increasing amount of our work centres around preventative care. I am conscious that I can order a test or prescribe a medicine and then move on, never realizing or knowing the effects of my decision. Each individual act is just part of a chain of events, a Mexican wave which gathers momentum as it unfolds.

So, coming back to John, how can I act as his advocate and be confident that his decision is an informed one? There is no perfect solution. The best case scenario may be to guarantee that he can talk to *me* (not *us*) about the decision on more than one occasion; to ask if he wants *me* to explain things to his daughter; to give him the assurance that we are in this together and that he is not just another NHS number. The anonymity which comes with our bureaucratic structures can't be reconciled with the mission statement of 'patient-centred care'.

Should I Have a Statin?

Ayesha Ahmed is a widow in her late 60s, generally fit and well, although her BP is a bit high and she has asthma. She has lots of friends, does charity work, and volunteers at the local Oxfam shop. Life is generally pretty good and she stays away from doctors as far as she can. As a result of her annual blood test, done because she has high BP, she has been offered a prescription of a statin to lower her cholesterol. This is because the risk algorithm we use has calculated that she has a 12 per cent chance of having a heart attack or stroke in the next ten years. The national guidelines recommend treatment with a statin, which will lower this risk to 8 or 9%.

She asks me if her cholesterol is very high. I tell her no, that it's similar to mine and is pretty normal. She is perplexed. I explain that the risk score is cumulative, based on all her risk factors including her age, ethnicity, and high BP. She asks whether changing her diet will help. I encourage her to eat healthily, which she does by and large in any case – but tell her it is unlikely that the treatment recommendation will change even if she does cut out ghee and her weekly bar of chocolate. Mrs. Ahmed is used to being proactive and to making any changes needed to keep her healthy. She isn't happy about this turn of events.

'Well', she asks, 'will it stop me having a stroke then?' I explain that I really don't know. I tell her that for every 1000 patients like her who are prescribed a statin, about eighteen will avoid having a heart attack or stroke over a period of five years because of it, that they would have had otherwise. She looks confused. 'What, so 982 wouldn't? Am I missing something?' I tell her no and that it's actually pretty good odds for a medicine used to prevent disease. 'And what about side effects?', she asks. I explain that treating her with a statin will slightly increase her risk of diabetes and may give her muscle pain. One of the difficulties is that the guideline is based on people *like* Ayesha. It doesn't take into account that Ayesha herself walks three miles every day, doesn't drink alcohol, and has a full life with a clear purpose and many friends – all of which are protective factors that are not accounted for.

'What I wonder is if I want to prevent a heart attack?', she says eventually. 'I mean, it isn't a bad way to go really, is it?' I agree

that in many ways, it isn't a bad way to go – staying well and then
having a big heart attack and knowing nothing more. I would
be tempted to choose this as an option for myself if I could also
determine the timing – so that it happens when I have lived for
a long time but not so long that I lose my faculties or become a
burden for my daughters. Perhaps if treated, Ayesha Ahmed will
live long enough because of the statin to get dementia or cancer,
like so many of my other patients. But then if I don't prescribe it,
what if instead of a fatal heart attack, she ends up having a stroke
which leaves her incapacitated?

These questions are unanswerable and I wonder if it is better
just to tell her what to do – make the decision that she doesn't
really need a statin and then code this as 'statin declined'. I don't
know what is best for her overall, only what is statistically most
likely to prolong her life.

'Your blood pressure is (still) above target.' We have been here
before.

Veronica Smith has had three text messages and two phone calls
from the practice asking her to come in and have her BP checked.
She is on the practice hypertension register and there are incentives
to measure and treat her BP to target. Unfortunately, it is not at
target, it is a bit raised. In the past, we have tried five different drugs
to lower it. They have been successful from my point of view, in
terms of the numbers. However, in different ways, they have all
made her feel ill and she has stopped taking them. The computer
predicts that she has a 20 per cent risk of having a heart attack
or stroke over the next ten years. If I successfully treat her blood
pressure, this risk will go down to 12 per cent. In theory. For people
like her. But how should I interpret this statistic for her in particular?

She is stressed out because she thinks her pension won't cover
her rent. Her husband has chronic back pain, is medically retired,
and she is now his carer. This is why she eventually agrees to
attend her BP check because he couldn't manage without her and
she knows she shouldn't neglect her health. She has told me that
she can't think of anything worse than living into her 90s but she
doesn't want to be left debilitated by a stroke. What should I advise
her? The BP medications I have prescribed before have left her
feeling tired, have given her swollen ankles, and have meant she
needed to get up at night to go to the loo. Is that worth the price of

possibly reducing her chance of having a stroke? How lucky is she feeling?

The other issue is that her high BP is inextricably linked to her social situation – the stress of living in poverty. There is increasing evidence that chronic stress (e.g., arising as a result of low socio-economic status) is linked to hypertension.[10] However, addressing stress does not feature in the NICE hypertension management guideline.[11] This feels ironic because I have a strong suspicion that if Veronica Smith wasn't constantly worried about being evicted, she might not need any drugs. Am I brave enough to put aside the decision about medication for now and instead ask her to see our social prescriber, with the rationale that reducing her stress will reduce her blood pressure, even if this is not in the guideline? The precise effect on BP of alleviating financial worry has not been as clearly quantified in trials as medication has been, since it is often pharmaceutical companies who fund the large, expensive trials which underpin evidence-based medicine.

In the end, I code her as 'BP treatment declined' and now there will be no more yellow triangles this year. And when they reappear next April, the scene will replay, with me in the role of the healthcare professional or maybe substituted with a different GP, pharmacist, or nurse.

People who actually want to see a GP have to spend time and effort navigating the system, waiting in long queues which are either digital or literal, and listening to endless background muzak in audio loops. The irony is that many patients who really don't want to be seen – those with risk factors for chronic disease for example – are pursued and cajoled into the surgery. Generally, people who value their lives are the ones who agree to attend.

In contrast, there are many 'unworried, unwell' who are heading towards premature deaths, who should be seen, but who will fall under the scrutiny of the medical gaze either too late or not at all. Their names will surface only when there is a call from the coroner, enquiring about when they were last seen by a doctor.

Diabetes Is a Social Disease

You are the same age as me, we both grew up in working-class neighbourhoods and we both have parents with diabetes. But that's where the similarity ends.

I have dodged my genetic destiny because my world now isn't the same as the one I grew up in, but yours is. Where I live, everybody exercises, avoids carbs, and does yoga – and it's catching. We all take self-preservation seriously. So I buy almonds and blueberries, avoid large portions and white bread. I walk or run, never take the bus. Work is interesting. I still feel young, even though I'm not. But in all ways apart from our chronological age, I am younger than you.

Because it's different for you. You don't matter to yourself as much as I do to me. Your extra weight means that you developed diabetes when you were still in your 30s, ten years ago. In the last decade, you have collected medications from me. You had to be persuaded to start the first one, but now you are a fully-fledged patient, on four different pills a day and an injection a week. To reduce your risk of dying or of an expensive major event like a heart attack or stroke.

Today, I am telling you that despite the four medicines and the injection, you are still failing at controlling your sugar. You are failing to muster the energy and finances you need to go to the gym, walk instead of taking the bus to work, and stop eating microwave meals. Maybe I can persuade you that things could be much better for you if you would care enough about yourself to change your ways. I can send you to the social prescriber, to the health coach, for subsidized exercise classes. But if you miss work, you don't get paid. And who will pick your grandkids up from school and look after them if you go for a workout? It's a nice thought, but these appointments are no good to you. So, instead, I will add another medicine to the mix. I can follow the guidelines and you can swallow another pill that might make you live a bit longer, or maybe not. And you accept what I tell you, and you will put up with the side effects because you don't have any choice.

I am wondering, as we talk, what my role is in this predicament – am I helping you with the cocktail I prescribe you or am I part of the system that has let you down? The root cause of this chronic disease is social,[12,13] not too much sugar and it could easily have been me sitting in your chair instead of you.

Talking about Pain

NICE's guideline 193 on chronic pain steers the discourse around this thorny subject.[14] It starts with semantics – whether to call pain that will not go away 'chronic' or 'persistent', a question that relates to which ideological position is adopted in the politics of pain. A guideline occupies an important position in these political conflicts – it is not just a battle of words, it is a statement about whose pain deserves to be alleviated and which methods of alleviation should be available on the NHS. For the first time, guideline 193 features qualitative syntheses of patient–clinician encounters and produces a checklist for good conversations about pain.

Talking about Pain – How Pain Affects Life and How Life Affects Pain

(Extract from NICE guideline 193)

Ask the person to describe how chronic pain affects their life, and that of their family, carers, and significant others, and how aspects of their life may affect their chronic pain.

- Lifestyle and day-to-day activities, including work and sleep disturbance;
- physical and psychological well-being;
- stressful life events, including previous or current physical or emotional trauma;
- current or past history of substance misuse;
- social interaction and relationships;
- difficulties with employment, housing, income, and other social concerns.

Be sensitive to the person's socio-economic, cultural and ethnic background, and faith group, and think about how these might influence their symptoms, understanding and choice of management.

Explore a person's strengths as well as the impact of pain on their life. This might include talking about:

- their views on living well;
- the skills they have for managing their pain;
- what helps when their pain is difficult to control.

Ask the person about their understanding of their condition, and that of their family, carers, and significant others. This might include:

• their understanding of the causes of their pain;
• their expectations of what might happen in the future in relation to their pain and their understanding of the outcome of possible treatments.[15]

The next two stories feature conversations about pain in the messy context of the consultation room – the habitat of street-level bureaucrats.

The Acceptance Dance – Scripts of Suffering

'It's killing me, doctor', says the woman. With difficulty, she rises from the chair in the waiting room and grunts on our joint way to the physiotherapy consulting room. She cannot make it to my room, as there are too many steps. I know she will have a lament, and this is exactly what I don't want to hear.[16] I would prefer something that I can fix, something that will be neatly finished with the sound of prescription paper exiting the printer as a reification of closure.

This will not happen. Her husband has come with her to support her case. He is the advocate. He is holding a piece of paper: the agenda. For now, he is holding on to it and won't give it to me yet – instead, he will play it later like the trump card in a game of whist. First, I have to listen.

'The shoulder man said I need to be referred to the Neurosurgeon', she says. 'It's getting worse.' I feel the vibes of suffering, the plea for respite from the pain that is grinding her down. This is only the second time I have met her. Her medical records are a list of one problem after another, and nothing ever works.

I am observing her movements, her facial expression, her hands, and her gaze, whilst listening to her lament. This performance asks a lot from me. I must restrain any attempt to speed the consultation up, to colonize her lament with words or supposedly easy solutions. I know there are no easy solutions and agreeing to what she brought up as an agenda item, 'refer to the Neurosurgeons' is one of these false shortcuts. I know for sure that there are no surgical options, the neurosurgeons will not be interested, and the Shoulder man was only trying to eject the problem into the nirwana of the waiting list, stuck in the mindset of surgery as the ultimate escalation step. The other steps include medication, the so-called analgesic ladder.

In this metaphor, she is already at the top. She takes Morphine and pregabalin, an anticonvulsant drug used to numb nerves, useful in epilepsy and nerve injuries.

I reply to her initial remark, 'This is not killing you. I think it is worse – you have to endure it'. Like successful torture, she endures the pain without dying, it is aimed to break her, and I think now she is at a point where her morale has been broken. I see this in her face, I hear it in her voice. She is desperate. This is a consultation at a breaking point.

At this moment her husband plays the trump card. 'Try zopiclone' (a sleeping tablet, related to Valium) and 'Increase her dose of pregabalin' are written on it.

I should not prescribe these drugs. I was part of the guideline development group that decided after studying all drug trials for chronic pain, that sleeping tablets and anticonvulsants of this class are not effective for chronic pain, or, from another paradigm, for ongoing suffering. The situation was uncomfortable. They were asking me for something that would not help – referral for surgery – and for something the guidelines tell me not to do – to give more medication. Medication that I know will not work and which might generate dependence.

A dilemma is a situation where there is no right outcome. Everything you do is wrong. Devil or deep blue sea, rock or hard place. This is a dilemma. I am still in acting mode. I would like to have an honest conversation with her without dismissing how she feels, and I am waiting for the right time.

I think that it would be wrong for me to refer her to a neurosurgeon, knowing for sure that it will not help, and will only cement her belief that the surgeon is the highest trump card in the symbolic order of suffering. I tell her that if I was a surgeon, I would not want to operate on her, because I would only operate if I thought that she would be better after surgery than before. I tell her that I feel this is more a case of unbearable suffering, and there is no medical cure.

Deep inside, I think 'put up with it'.

A now retired colleague, loved by her patients but blunt in her utterances used to say it. 'Put up with it.' She said it to colleagues when they complained about workload, and she said it also to patients. She had a reputation for being kind.

'Put up with it.' I tell her what I am thinking and that I know it is a brutal thought. Now we are in the game. She says that she has had so much pain for so long, all her life, and all she does is put up with it; for years and years. And sometimes putting up with it works. At these times, my colleagues and I will not see her. Chronic pain is not chronic; it is not a monotonous state of affairs, but it is a dramatic space with ups and downs. We have met today in the here and now of a down, at a breaking point. She says that she has a high pain threshold, but the last few nights have simply been too much.

She just wants to sleep. 'Just' – every time I hear the word 'just' in these situations I know it is asking the impossible. She wants a respite from the pain. One good night. A pit stop of being without pain, knowing well that she will return to the pain that lasts forever, that has become part of her life.

She mentions her brittle bones that do not hold screws and her other unresolved problems. 'Do you think I have Fibromyalgia?', she asks.

I invite her in for a thorough assessment. 'Rather than sending you away, I would like to get to know you better', I say and book her for an extended consultation with me. I decide to invest my time, knowledge, and energy in her.

'I am sorry, we are going to Scotland on a mini-break', she replies.

What a paradigm change.

I say that I don't think that the sleeping tablets and pregabalin are helpful in the long run, but if they ease the work of putting up with it, I will do what I should not do and prescribe in the short term.

I press 'print' and the sound of the printer provides closure of yet another episode of pain.

She did not come back for the extended consultation.

Words That Hurt, Words That Heal

George, the trainee, sent me a message on WhatsApp to say that a telephone consultation had gone wrong, so he had booked the patient in with me in two days' time. It had been a long consultation about which painkillers to use to kill the patient's pain. He had asked whether she could instead 'suck it up' (painkillers are no longer recommended as a treatment of choice in guidelines on pain management). It is what doctors sometimes think but don't say aloud. He told me that he immediately realized that it was the wrong thing to say, that he had hurt her feelings – but there was no way to back track. She said she never wanted to see him again and wanted me to have a professional conversation with him about the kind of language that should be used in clinical encounters.

So, we arranged to meet – in the physiotherapy room, as she cannot climb the stairs to my consulting room.

We had met twice before, and the first consultation had been challenging and memorable. She disclosed then that she had been systematically and repeatedly raped by her own father. She talked about the numerous hurtful interactions she had subsequently had with healthcare professionals. She mentioned the gynaecologist who for religious reasons did not want to treat her when she read the label 'termination of pregnancy' in her notes. The doctor did not enquire further, so she did not hear that the baby would have been both a child and sibling for the patient.

During the second consultation, we talked about the role of her medication, dihydrocodeine, which belongs to the opiate family, a few steps down from morphine. We both felt that it wasn't helping the pain itself and that it may have created a new problem – dependency. We agreed that she should carefully reduce and then stop it, and I referred her to a psychologically informed service that specializes in weaning people off prescription drugs.

Trainee George happened to be the one who had to conduct the subsequent conversation with her about what to do instead, now that the decision had been made to discontinue dihydrocodeine. His foray into the possibility of living without painkillers when they clearly don't do what they should do – kill the pain – ended catastrophically.

The patient and her advocate sat in front of me in the physiotherapy room and explained how disgusted they were with George's choice of words – 'suck it up'. How could he say such things to a victim of sexual abuse – or to anyone? It ripped open all the old wounds. It is what her father had said to her. It is what she heard all the time. The disbelief came back, the shame, the hurt.

Words can hurt.

We talked about what to do with the trainee and how to teach him to choose words wisely, particularly in interactions with traumatized people.

But we also came back to her dilemma: after having successfully ended the relationship with dihydrocodeine, a problem remained. What should she do about her back pain? She clearly needed something, or should she just go on like this forever? She is only in her 50s, how can she have a meaningful future in this state? She asked for a scan, she wanted to establish the state of her spine – the 'end organ' as they call it in pain medicine. We talked a bit about brains and end organs, but most of the words came from me.

I felt that at this moment the conversation was in a very difficult phase. I had to be tender, while also addressing the brutal question of how to live with pain that will not go away, and how to approach the 'always' and 'forever' with acceptance. I chose not to answer straight away and more importantly to create an atmosphere in

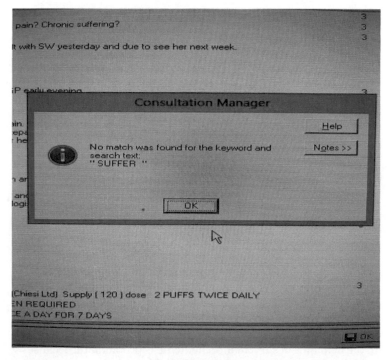

FIGURE 3.2: 'Suffer is not a recognised diagnosis'. It is not recognized by the clinical IT system. Jens Foell, 2021.

which acceptance could be an option. Silence with eye contact was what I was aiming for. But inside, I was thinking, 'Yes, the pain will be there forever' (or other versions of the suck-it-up trope) and I could not look her in the eye. So instead, I said, 'Of course nobody can say forever or always – things change'.

But we both knew that her life will continue to consist of living with pain. Our task now was to find ways of trying to alleviate this, to take the edge off. We ended the consultation with an agreement to increase the dose of the antidepressant she takes, which may or may not have an effect on her pain experience, and with me inviting her to have acupuncture, to see if it helps and if it is a tool she can adapt to use herself.

These stories highlight the delicate conversations about acceptance of chronic pain and the subtle differences between pain and suffering.

Reflection

As in the field of law, and as the stories in this chapter demonstrate, there is a tension between the letter of the guideline and its spirit – the dialectic of bureaucracy. The spirit of the guideline is nebulous though. Documented decisions are difficult to criticize using an elusive spirit, they are easy to criticize using the letter of the law. An unintended consequence has been that 'application of social power through the model of scientific bureaucratic medicine has altered the conception of what it is to be a doctor – especially a general practitioner'.[17]

Within a scientific bureaucratic paradigm, GPs are conceptualized as enactors of guidelines. This assumes that patients present with well-defined, single illnesses that can be directly related to the evidence. It is at odds with the lived experience of GPs where each individual encounter is unique and where the underlying cause of the disease is multifactorial. There is tension in applying generic rules to contexts for which they were not designed. Healthcare workers commonly face a conflict of priority between listening to the patient and listening to the demands of surveillance medicine. This is the uncomfortable decision-making space of *street-level bureaucrats*.[18] Listening to the demands of surveillance medicine is problematic because guidelines generally refer to individual diseases rather than to people with multiple illnesses. For some people, it means that the burden of adverse effects caused by preventative medicine and the intrusion of frequent surveillance appointments is worse than the burden of their medical condition. Underlying social determinants of health are usually ignored in guidelines, as is the co-occurrence of illnesses like diabetes and depression, which are often driven by social factors such as poor housing and financial stress. Emily Mendenhall, in her book *Rethinking Diabetes*, uses the term 'syndemic' to describe this phenomenon. Arguably, a syndemic framework would be better suited to primary care than single disease guidelines.[12]

The rise of the scientific bureaucratic paradigm has been made possible by technology – computers that are used to record and monitor activity levels. The requirement to fill in templates with pre-structured digitalized interfaces has become entirely embedded so that it is now part of the identity of clinicians working in general practice.

Computers are no longer adjuncts, but active participants in the consultation, able to influence which questions are asked and what is prioritized.[19] In reality, clinicians are as much in dialogue with the computer as they are with the patient. Likewise, patients are also in an invisible dialogue with guidelines and algorithms. We might wonder who is doing the talking within the consultation and how 'meaning' is generated in a coherent way between the three protagonists.[20]

Algorithms used in managing patients' access and flow through the system are informed by research evidence. Once used in the informational infrastructure of decision-making systems, it is impossible to go 'under' these foundations. Clinicians and patients must negotiate the dissonance between 'like me' and 'me' – the difference between the macro-level of population averages, taking into account over- or under-representation of particular subgroups (e.g., in terms of age, ethnicity, social deprivation, etc.) and the micro-level of the individuals involved in the encounter. It is a space of uncertainty. The sociologist David Armstrong comments that power lies with the paradigm that dominates it.[21]

When considering the space of uncertainty, it is worth noting that there is a growing body of evidence about the tacit way in which decisions are made in real life.[22] 'Mindlines' is a term that has been used to describe 'guidelines-in-the-head' which clinicians create for themselves over time, based on data from different sources, practical experience, and contextual factors. These mindlines are used to inform decision-making – and may be as important as written guidelines in informing evidence-based practice. Studies have shown that mindlines are affected and changed by discussions with colleagues.[23] The implication is that the culture of the practice and the conversations which take place within it influence how guidelines are applied in real life.

Notes

1. Paul Kalanithi, *When Breath Becomes Air* (Random House, 2016).

2. Archibald Leman Cochrane, *Effectiveness and Efficiency: Random Reflections on Health Services* (London: Nuffield Trust, 1972).

3. Julian Tudor Hart, 'The Inverse Care Law', *The Lancet* 297, no. 7696 (1971): 405–12.

4. 'Introduction to the Principles of Morals and Legislation', 1907, http://www.laits.utexas.edu/poltheory/bentham/ipml/index.html.

5. Franco Sassi, 'Calculating QALYs, Comparing QALY and DALY Calculations', *Health policy and planning* 21, no. 5 (2006): 402–08.

6. Stefan Timmermans and Steven Epstein, 'A World of Standards but Not a Standard World: Toward a Sociology of Standards and Standardization', *Annual Review of Sociology* 36, no. 1 (2010): 69–89.

7. Geoffrey C. Bowker and Susan Leigh Star, *Sorting Things Out: Classification and Its Consequences* (Cambridge, MA: MIT Press, 2000).

8. Donald A. Schön, *Educating the Reflective Practitioner: Toward a New Design for Teaching and Learning in the Professions* (San Francisco, CA: Jossey-Bass, 1987).

9. David Haslam, 'Getting the Guidance Right', 2016, accessed December 23, 2022, https://www.nice.org.uk/news/feature/david-haslam-getting-the-guidance-right.

10. Tanya M. Spruill, 'Chronic Psychosocial Stress and Hypertension', *Current Hypertension Reports* 12, no. 1 (2010): 10–16.

11. NICE, *NICE Clinical Guideline 136. Hypertension Diagnosis and Management in Adults* (2022).

12. Emily Mendenhall. *Rethinking Diabetes: Entanglements with Trauma, Poverty, and Hiv* (Ithaca, NY: Cornell University Press, 2019).

13. The Marmot Review, *Fair Society, Healthy Lives: The Marmot Review. Strategic Review of Health Inequalities in England Post-2010* (UCL Institute of Health Equity, 2010), http://www.parliament.uk/documents/fair-society-healthy-lives-full-report.pdf.

14. Serena Carville, Margaret Constanti, Nick Kosky, Cathy Stannard, and Colin Wilkinson, 'Chronic Pain (Primary and Secondary) in over 16s: Summary of NICE Guidance', *BMJ* 373 (2021): n895.

15. Keith Wailoo, 'Thinking through the Pain', *Perspectives in Biology and Medicine* 59, no. 2 (2016): 253–62.

16. B. Bub, 'The Patient's Lament: Hidden Key to Effective Communication: How to Recognise and Transform', *Medical humanities* 30, no. 2 (2004): 63–69.

17. George Hull and Sally Hull, 'Recovering General Practice from Epistemic Disadvantage', in *Person-centred Primary Care*, ed. C Dowrick (New York: Routledge, 2017).

18. Michael Lipsky, *Street-Level Bureaucracy: Dilemmas of the Individual in Public Service* (Thousand Oaks, CA: Russell Sage Foundation, 2010).

19. Deborah Swinglehurst, Celia Roberts, and Trisha Greenhalgh, 'Opening up the "Black Box" of the Electronic Patient Record: A Linguistic Ethnographic Study in General Practice', *Communications Medicine* 8, no. 1 (2011): 3–15.

20. Rupal Shah, Robert Clarke, Sanjiv Ahluwalia, and John Launer, 'Finding Meaning in the Consultation: Introducing the Hermeneutic Window', *British Journal of General Practice* 70, no. 699 (2020): 502–03.

21. David Armstrong, 'Actors, Patients and Agency: A Recent History', *Sociology of Health & Illness* 36, no. 2 (2014): 163–74.

22. Malin Andre, Lars Borgquist, Mats Foldevi, and Sigvard Mölstad, 'Asking for "Rules of Thumb": A Way to Discover Tacit Knowledge In General Practice', *Family Practice* 19, no. 6 (2002): 617–22.

23. John Gabbay and Andrée le May, 'Mindlines: Making Sense of Evidence in Practice', *British Journal of General Practice* 66 (2016): 402–03.

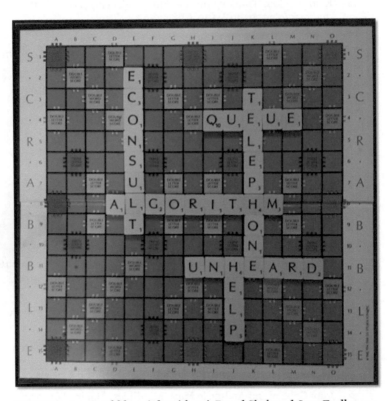

FIGURE 4.1: Scrabble 4, 'Algorithms', Rupal Shah and Jens Foell, 2021.

4.
Waiting to Connect: Algorithms That Dictate Access

*Consider the objects we use, the food we eat, and how
the experiences we have are mostly mass-produced and
packaged in remote factories. Commodification follows.
Commercialisation opportunistically enters as a siren, the
dominant force. This, increasingly, is our world [...] remotely
sourced, generated and controlled.[1]*
> (David Zigmond, former GP and Psychiatrist, London)

*I feel disconnected, alienated and fearful whilst delivering
services over the phone to people with similar disconnected
and sensory limitations.*
> (Jens – recovering from COVID-19, July 2021)

From 'Go with the Flow' to Demand Management
War is the mother of invention. Life is a battlefield. Maybe it is
fitting that 'triage', the term used to categorize the wounded has its
origins in the Napoleonic wars.[2]

Nineteenth-century war medicine needed to prioritize urgent
medical care for battle casualties, in order to most effectively
direct inadequate resources at a time when demand vastly
outstripped supply. This resulted in the categorization of injuries
into different levels of severity, which were assigned their own
frames of response. Since those days, the career of *triage* as
a way of sorting workload prior to doing the work has soared
to new heights, so it is no longer confined only to emergency
medicine but also features in routine healthcare. It is justified

97

by the scarcity paradigm, which assumes that resources can never match demand – something that seems incontrovertible, although it has been challenged.[3,4]

To an extent, when working within bureaucratic systems, the scarcity paradigm becomes a self-fulfilling prophecy. This is because there is an underlying assumption that all human maladies can and should be slotted into categories and thus incorporated into protocols and from there into pathways (see 'Pigeonholes' for more on this topic). It results in a belief amongst politicians, clinicians, and patients that medical coverage should be all-encompassing.[5] The obvious answer is endless expansion, with more and more services and complicated referral pathways set up to deal with the apparently increasing demand, which it could be argued is self-generated. And demand must be managed somehow, so the questions 'What is urgent?' and 'What is an emergency?' appear with unwavering regularity in every meeting in services that are underfunded and over-stretched. The management of waiting lists, queues, and access is bound up with organizational hierarchies. The call for standardization and uniformity (and fairness around access) is therefore loud!

Coming back to triage, primary care physicians are trained to use their generalist skills for patients presenting with undifferentiated health problems – that is, anyone who walks through the door, with any problem. But people are now discouraged from just walking through the door; and 'undifferentiatedness' is increasingly rare in contemporary healthcare.

'GIRFT' is the acronym standing for the most efficient Hogwarts-sorting hat: 'GET IT RIGHT FIRST TIME'. 'Right clinician at the right time for the right condition.' The ultimate sweet spot. Bull's Eye. Most differentiation work is now done by algorithms in conjunction with their human operators in various ratios of control and command between the human and the machine component of the man/machine chimera. The ability to override the rules of the algorithm depends on professional seniority. The algorithm is particularly prominent in Out-of-Hours (OoH) services compared to in-hours practice access. Readers who have used NHS 111 will be very familiar with it. The standardization generates fidelity in the assessment process. Call handlers MUST follow the script. Their key performance indicators include adherence to protocol. If something goes wrong in the process, workers are safe if they demonstrate that they have followed the script. Their role is to be the human side of the man/machine chimera. Their boss is indeed the algorithm, and the organizational hierarchy curates this set of rules.

Healthcare professionals spend lots of time memorizing mental checklists for the conditions that form their workload, so they remember to ask the right questions and consider alternative diagnoses. Information technology enables these checklists to be built into platforms that mediate contact with callers. In the field of triage, there is a long-standing debate about who should make decisions about which patients get prioritized to receive treatment most urgently: should a senior person with years of clinical experience make decisions, or can a lack of experience be substituted or augmented by sets of rules? In the analogy of airline safety systems, should the pilot be in charge, or the assisting system? What are the power relationships about overriding one or the other? Boeing's fatal crashes arose when the 'auto-pilot' was in charge, and the pilots could not override the new system. Auto-pilot proved to be fatal.[6] The man/machine chimera can be an untrustworthy creature. This is a real-life example of NHS 111 prose taken from a general practice (GP) OoH shift, illustrating the way meaning can be lost when interpreted through an algorithm and treatment might therefore at best be misdirected and at worst, dangerous:

> Advanced Duplicate Calls: No Duplicates Found based on probability parameters Advanced Duplicate Calls: No Duplicates Found based on probability parameters W3W Reverse Lookup For Current Location: unclaimed.opens.ribs Pre-Enter Detail [...] Is the Patient Awake?: Yes Is the Patient Breathing?: Yes What's The Problem: **M-CLOTS,HEAD FEELS LIKE EXPLOADING,ITCHING** Advanced Duplicate Calls: No Duplicates Found based on probability parameters PT DUE TO SEE DERMATOLOGIST ON THE 16TH BUT UNABLE TO COPE TILL THEN PT HAS MARKS ALL OVER HIS BODY – RASH LIKE CLOTS ALL OVER HIM – UNWELL What's The Problem: **M-CLOTS,HEAD FEELS LIKE EXPLOADING,ITCHING** Advanced Duplicate Calls: No Duplicates Found based on probability parameters Party (ProQA): 2nd Party Caller Crew Responder Information (ProQA): 64-year-old, Male, Conscious, Breathing. Caller Statement: **M-CLOTS,HEAD FEELS**

LIKE EXPLOADING,ITCHING Advanced Duplicate Calls: No Duplicates Found based on probability parameters **PT BLEEDING ON HIS HEAD HE'S SCRATCHING SO MUCH** ProQA:URGENT:Only one COVID-related symptom identified by EIDS Tool evaluation – proceed with caution. User Comments (ProQA): **ALL OVER HIS BODY – ESPECIALLY ON HIS HEAD** Party (ProQA): 2nd Party Caller ProQA CAD Response: GREEN3 ProQA CBRN [...] CBRN: COVID Tool ? only ONE symptom identified ? proceed with caution >received a COVID vaccination >chills Key Questions (ProQA): 1. He is completely alert (responding appropriately). 2. He is breathing normally. 3. He is not bleeding (or vomiting blood). 4. He has other pain: **ALL OVER HIS BODY – ESPECIALLY ON HIS HEAD** 5. No priority symptoms (ALPHA conditions 2–12 not identified). 6. His primary problem is itching. 7. The EMD launched the EIDS Tool. 8. Only one COVID-related symptom identified. User Comments (ProQA): **ALL OVER HIS BODY – ESPECIALLY ON HIS HEAD** Party (ProQA): ((Health Advisor) (Wales))

HCP / RASH / ONGOING AND WORSENING / MILD LIGHT SENSITIVITY / HEADACHE 2 DAYS / PS 8/10

RASH / SKIN LUMPS 1 YEAR +

UNDER CARE OF GP AND REFERRED TO DERM – AWAITING APP

RASH WORSENING LAST 2 DAYS – IS SPREADING

JUST COMPLETED COURSE OF ABX

Apart from war, *necessity* is also a mother of invention (and innovation). The physical distancing requirements of healthcare delivery during COVID-19 restrictions boosted developments such as web-based triage and remote consultations that were already in the process of being introduced at large scale in primary and secondary care – and allowed them to be implemented without being backed up by evidence from large, controlled trials. The COVID-19-generated lockdown ended any lingering doubts about the lack of evidence and positioned primary care firmly into the new world of 'total triage', enshrined in binding service stipulations. The writing was already on the wall – even before COVID-19, the NHS Long Term Plan[7] which was published in 2019 stated, '*In ten years' time, we expect the existing model of care to look markedly different. The NHS will offer a "digital first" option for most'.*

Many private companies offer their services to help healthcare services manage demand virtually, using programmes which are often the product of a collaboration between clinicians and software developers. Selecting which data is used as a source for the software and determining how often the triage assistance programmes are updated and to what extent they are responsive to local requirements varies from provider to provider. These systems do not use artificial intelligence – there is no automatic learning from service data and population data built into the algorithms. Maintenance and update are subject to the contractual arrangements between purchasing and provider organizations – money matters.

Triage assistance/flow management programmes are multidimensional instruments. As well as dictating/assisting decisions about patient flow, they also capture data about patients' interactions with operators (i.e., the call handlers, triage clinicians, or clinicians completing the task) and therefore can be used to measure key performance indicators (KPIs). Adherence to triage rules and time taken per call by triage clinicians are examples. But the outputs used are snapshots and do not give information about the turbulences and roadblocks in patients' 'journeys' as service-users. It is ironic, since it is the patient's experiences of the twists and turns in their passage through the system which matters most. This information cannot be easily drawn from the dataset. The mantra is 'you will only need to tell your story once' but, of course, that is a fallacy, as stories are more than data capture points. The repurposing of stories in this way can inadvertently de-legitimize the patient's voice (see also 'Pigeonholes').[8]

Many GP surgeries now use form-based online triage systems such as 'e-consult' (eConsult Health Ltd) which require patients to fill in details about their symptoms as well as other information such as smoking status and alcohol consumption. Practice teams respond to these forms – with anything from a text message to a telephone consultation or an offer of a face-to-face appointment. But some clinicians prefer to avoid face-to-face consultations, which require the interaction to be processed in emotional as well as cognitive mode. When a problem is presented as a disease category, it enables a response which is purely cognitive with less emotional burden on the practitioner.

A headache on a form is simple, linear, and logical. There are clear guidelines which can be applied. This is in contrast to a real person with a headache, whose pain might be multifactorial and might not go away unless the underlying trigger (stress at work, an unhappy relationship, domestic violence, economic uncertainty, etc.) is addressed. Since it is so much simpler, the temptation is to treat the form-based representation of the symptom, particularly in time-pressured settings (see 'The Bad Mother' later in this chapter). Indeed, some clinicians prefer the neatness of the story represented as data capture points, which can be processed remotely, whilst simultaneously navigating the internet for guidelines and additional support. Whilst others prefer to be exposed to the blood, sweat, and tears of the patient in front of them.

Interactions which take the presenting symptom at face value can send patients down rabbit holes of pointless investigations and treatments. People may re-consult time and again until the clinician gets it right. This generates an artificially high volume of demand, with clinicians going down routes that lead down blind alleys. Platform-mediated triage which relies on disease categorization might ultimately add to demand on the health service and to workload because it fails to take into account the difference between 'disease' and the way in which patients actually experience ill health.[9,10] The increase in ambulance calls and ED utilization after the gradual easing of lockdown rules adds weight to this suspicion,[11] although it is clear that the bottleneck in service provision is influenced by many other factors, such as hospital throughput, discharge arrangements, and availability of community resources. The whole system is over-stretched.

No specialist in healthcare manufacturing has ever calculated the time it takes to deal with the friction that is such a fundamental part of contemporary healthcare, with its heavy reliance on information capture and processing on different platforms. Despite the rhetoric of joined-up care, seamless transition of care, robust services, and care wrapped around the patient, the recipients of such care describe their experience of service provision as fragmented and disrupted and feel they are 'lost in transit'. Clinical correspondence between the hospital and GP resembles a game of rumours. Letters take weeks to get to the GP and when they do, often fail to reflect the patient's experience of hospital, giving only coded diagnoses and

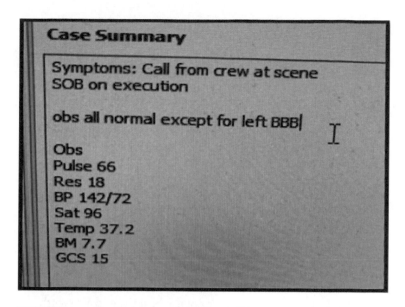

FIGURE 4.2: Confusing correspondence: 'SOB on execution'. Jens Foell, 2021.

medications or representations of the triage sequence. The gaps between services as they are imagined and services as they really are is huge. In fact, the lived experience of service provision can be summarized as 'wicked'.[12]

In this chapter, the stories are about flow – the flow of patients through a turbulent, over-stretched system in which access and response are often controlled by an algorithm and are increasingly remote, literally and metaphorically. Trying to manage health at arm's length using descriptions of symptoms on a form or via an algorithm can create turbulence, inefficiencies, and confusion.

The Tip of the Iceberg
'Shoot me!', said the beetle.

She sat on the comfy chair in her bungalow. Everything around her looked spotless and clean and so did she. I liked her straight away.

'Just shoot me!'

'Give me an injection!'

Her close relatives had driven up to look after her. Her house was crowded with them and us, two GPs visiting her.

Her son and daughter-in-law were there. It was the daughter-in-law who had called the GP OoH service, now under new management – NHS 111. The case had come up in the blue column, indicating that the algorithm recommended that the timeframe for call back should be two hours. 'Needs another prescription for antibiotics' was the headline. But the blurb beneath suggested that there was more to the story than 'needs another prescription', that what I saw was not what I would get.

I called, promised the prescription, and conveyed curiosity about the bigger picture. The daughter-in-law told me that her mother-in-law had become helpless – she needed carers at night, everything hurt, and she could not get up anymore, with consequences for bladder and bowel management. She had a pressure sore at the bottom of the spine and needed more dressings.

I asked whether it would help to visit to explore the bigger picture. Of course, Saturdays are not the best time to act swiftly on a dramatic increase in care needs. The family were grateful and surprised to receive a visit. I thought it was warranted despite the simple task, 'needs another prescription for antibiotics', but it was an unusual decision. Unlike the call handlers, GPs in OoH used to have at least some ability to apply discretion. This is less so now that they can no longer choose to pick up calls from their local area.

GP trainee Tamara was with me. We entered the room, the stage. The stage was set up for a drama. The drama was about how to deal with the impending end of an era. 'This last year has been difficult – in and out of hospital.' 'We did not expect her to be so poorly.' Tamara commented on the fact that the blurb presented to us about the reason for contacting the OoH service was only the tip of the iceberg. Underneath the water level could be found a decline in function over the last year, frequent infections, dramatically reduced mobility, and ultimately a woman now bed bound and dependent on others for the simplest tasks, like holding a beaker. She was very frail and very weak.

The son and daughter-in-law were understanding and in contrast to other relatives in similar situations, they did not convey anger and blame. I felt relieved. I could breathe. I had space.

Tamara and I examined, assessed, and orientated ourselves. The small talk was, as always, the source of important information. We heard that she had been the wife of a Reverend. That she had been very active in the community until recently, but the new turn of events had rendered her helpless.

'Just shoot me', she said. To me, she looked like a beetle on its back. So frail, so vulnerable, so delicate, so dependent on others, possibly so frustrated that this had happened to her, the proud person who used to be a help-giver rather than a help-receiver.

We could have a fluent, coherent, humorous, and sophisticated conversation. 'Give me the injection!', she repeated.

'Of course, I can't do this, don't want to do it, and am not allowed to do it. It would be murder. Not an option. Never ever.'

We sat at the table. An improvised best-interest-meeting. I wondered, 'is this the right time to do some straight talking? To mention the D word?'

I thought, 'how would she like doctors to deal with her heart when her time is up, if she dies?'

(I must say I came prepared. I had the Do Not Attempt Cardiopulmonary Resuscitation – DNACPR-form in my doctor's bag. I knew that this needs to be discussed in such a situation, where someone is about to need a more intensive care package.)

'She certainly would not want to be resuscitated!', said the son.

There was a long, but meaningful silence.

'We did not expect this conversation right now.'

I moved on and filled in the documentation, the paper with the red frame that needs to be left with the patient.

I called Social Services. I organized the padded dressing. I gave another prescription for antibiotics for a urine infection. The son told me about his work that takes him to people's houses. He said he repairs appliances and is familiar with the debris of families' clothes in washing machines.

I could promise him that his mother's care needs would be dealt with as a matter of urgency.

A week later, I called the patient back. I was directed to an answering machine, so I called the other number mentioned on the recorded message, belonging to the neighbour.

'Ah, you! Yes. On Thursday she was transferred to a nursing home, and on Friday she passed away. The son and daughter-in-law will come back later to deal with matters.'

In retrospect, it turned out that the blurb I was first presented with obscured the view under the tip of the iceberg. The matter at hand was a discussion about death and not about another prescription.

Is Lovesickness a Sickness? - Palpitations In Unscheduled Care

On service operation protocols, all work tasks allocated to me (Jens) when I work in GP OoH are controlled and vetted by a triage nurse. This nurse operates 60 miles away in a triage hub.

My caregiving micro-environment includes a minor injury unit and the ward of a cottage hospital. District nurses have their offices in the same building. We all talk to each other.

A District Nurse hijacks my room (bypassing my pimp, the triage call handler/algorithm-chimera) and expresses concern about Mrs. W, a new resident in a nearby supported living institution.

I know which room she lives in. I treated its previous resident who passed away there two weeks ago.

The District Nurse is concerned about Mrs. W's concern about her rapid heartbeat. She wonders whether she should call an ambulance, or get an ECG – the works.

I say that I wonder whether, in fact, the fast pulse is a symptom of anxiety – and rather than firing a battery of biomedical questions over the phone, I ask whether she, the nurse, might go to see Mrs. W and simply listen to her story.

This is what she does, and then she asks me to visit too, 'to cover my back'.

The patient has a Polish name. I speculate that she might have been transferred from the Polish village on Llyn Peninsula. This peculiar dwelling has been a Polish enclave since the end of the Second World War, constituted of decommissioned army barracks. There used to be a Catholic Polish church and a Polish library there.

But last year, support was withdrawn. The care home (run by nuns!) had to close. The residents were dispersed to other care homes. Many died, some of stress and broken hearts. I used to love visiting the Polish village and listening to the stories the residents told. It was a very peculiar place, out of kilter with its Welsh environment.

Mrs. W's story fits this theme. Sadly, it is a story of loss and displacement. Her partner is English and did not live in the Polish village, so he could not visit her during the COVID-19 lockdown. He developed dementia while they were separated by the virus, and it transpires that she is grieving for the personality that has evaded him already. He is bombarding her now with more than 60 phone calls per day. She feels guilty for wishing that he will die soon because this state is unbearable.

Several of her fellow community members died swiftly after having been dispersed.

She must settle into her new environment. She is 92, hard of hearing, and blind in one eye.

And all of this makes her upset. She is upset that she is not coping. Or that she might not cope. It is too early to tell.

Of course, an ambulance for her fast pulse is not the answer. But on paper it IS the answer. Medical causes need to be excluded. It is not safe to state, 'this physical abnormality is the manifestation of an emotional reaction to stressful circumstances' 60 miles away over the phone, without having a plausible alternative interpretation based on biography and circumstances rather than biological abnormalities.

I doubt there are questions about what is troubling her heart in the algorithm for dealing with a rapid pulse rate.

There is also little space for listening during a telephone triage encounter with a call centre 60 miles away, where the call handler – the person trained up to operate the algorithm machine – does not know, and might not be curious about the Polish Village, sister Beata, the Polish army and their dealings with the British Army during and after the Second World War, the Polish communities and their cohesion throughout the post-war and post-communist eras.

But this is what we talked about. And it made sense for her. Her pulse slowed down. The fear diminished. It was more a matter of pastoral care than a matter of 'escalation', which on paper it could have been.

On a similar note, I was called to deal with the high blood pressure of a resident in a nearby dementia care home. The blood pressure was unusually high, and the care home staff became anxious. Their written protocol dictated escalation. This meant phoning NHS 111, and the outcome of this escalation was to ask the GP, me, for a home visit.

The home visit changed the 'unusually high blood pressure needing medical escalation' to an expected physiological reaction to emotive life events: he told me that two days ago, he had attended his wife's funeral. And he did not know where this leaves him.

Remote triage leaves very little space for biographical explanations, which look negligent in the space of protocol. Alternative interpretations can be accepted only AFTER real, medical pathology has been excluded. This is a safe option. But this option comes at a price: the two people in this story would have had to travel to the District General Hospital and join the queue in Accident and Emergency, where they would eventually have been seen and then very likely returned to sender, after a treacherous journey back and forth. This is the price for playing it safe, with the normative biomedical interpretation paradigm in the dominant position.

These two stories are linked by the physical symptoms of lovesickness. Is lovesickness a disease? Do the vomiting, weight loss, fast pulse, high blood pressure, inability to focus, and to cope after an emotional injury warrant a full medical workup?

In the Loop

She walks in heavily, very slowly, shoulders hunched, dressed in multiple unmatching layers of jumpers, with a big, shapeless coat over them all. She smells of stale cigarettes and misery.

When she starts speaking, her speech is also very slow and slurred, as though she is drugged, which she is – by us, the medical profession.

'I ... am ... stuck ... in ... a ... loop', she says, looking down.

She has been discharged from the community mental health team (CMHT) because she hasn't got better and also hasn't got worse. She is 34 years old and has been bouncing back and forth to them for years. There is an alert on her notes saying 'Complex patient. Double appointments please'.

Her last psychiatry appointment was done remotely, by video. It was dysfunctional. When she said she might shoot herself, they asked where she would get a gun. She spent the rest of the evening exploring options.

She can't access the community self-referral cognitive behavioural therapy (CBT) service because her mental health is too bad, and she is too complex, but there isn't provision for her to have specialist therapy for her emotionally unstable personality disorder and recurrent depression.

'I ... am ... so ... lonely', she says. 'Nobody ... likes ... me, even ... I ... don't ... like ... me.'

'What is left? ... Where ... can ... you ... send ... me ... to ... get ... help?'

The letter from the CMHT says she wants to talk about the trauma of her childhood. They have suggested she buys a book on the subject and gets in touch with a charity that might be able to find her a befriender.

Without thinking, I ask her whether she wants to talk about it to me. To maybe start with the first ten years of her life.

She looks taken aback.

'Dr. Shah, whhattt whattt would be the pppppurpose of that?'

I am feeling very exposed now and fumbling, not sure where this is going. We are entering unchartered, forbidden territory with unexploded landmines hidden just under the surface, which I am not equipped to defuse.

I look directly at her. 'I hope it would help you to find some kind of meaning, and an explanation for what you are going through now and why you feel like this. But I don't know. I am not sure where I can send you, so I am offering you myself.' And then it's like a tap has been turned on. Her speech isn't slow any more, it's at a normal pace and fluent, and she is looking at me for the first time.

'Nobody has said that before.'

It comes spilling down like an avalanche. Her dad dying when she was 4, her mother leaving her behind in the Philippines to work abroad, living with an aunt who didn't like her, getting beaten for not doing tasks around the house as she should have, a predatory uncle, coming to the United Kingdom aged 12 to live with a mum she didn't know any more and who withheld her love. She says she started to steal money and use it to buy cigarettes, the more the better. She became addicted to them.

She is crying. I am too.

Then as quick as it started, the tap turns off. She gets up to go without being asked, takes my hand and thanks me and walks out of the room.

This scenario is commonly encountered in GP – where the most vulnerable patients are unable to access specialist services and are bounced from pillar to post, failing to receive the help they need.

A Blocked Nose

'Well, I wonder whether you have any idea of how to help me, Dr. Shah, because I don't mean to be rude, but I'm really fed up with getting text messages advising me to buy nose sprays and antihistamines when I contact the surgery.' I am working from home, sitting at the kitchen table because my 13-year-old has taken over the study for her home school lessons – secondary schools haven't re-opened yet. We are a few months into the first lockdown of 2020 and as restrictions start to ease, I am disorientated, not sure what lies ahead for the practice where I have worked for sixteen years. My husband wanders across to make himself a drink and I try to make sense of what Mr. Sidwell is saying over the drone of the coffee machine. I can see his notes on my laptop until I lose connection to the practice computer system. I wish I had read the last few consultations more thoroughly before I called him, but at least I know him well.

Mr. Sidwell is a widower in his 70s. He often says that he is a 'coper', which seems plausible, though before COVID-19 he came to the surgery every couple of weeks with a new complaint. He was always cleanly shaven and sported a blazer, shirt, and tie. 'Well, how are *you* keeping?', he would ask, leaning forward, concerned, giving me the impression that it was I who had come to consult him.

Back to the kitchen table.

'Hang on, I can't see your notes. Can we rewind a bit? What's been happening?'

'Well, my hay fever is ridiculous, quite frankly. I just can't go out, I'm totally trapped in the house.'

I rack my brain. Of all the different things I have seen him for, I am pretty sure that hay fever isn't one.

'When did you develop hay fever? I'm sorry but I didn't realize you have it.'

'Well, I didn't before this, it's quite new. And the medicines I've been prescribed have been next to useless I'm afraid. Oh well,

I suppose I shall have to weather out the storm indoors for the foreseeable.' He sighs with such exaggerated exasperation that I think he is on the verge of hanging up.

'Well, let's at least see if there's something that can be done about it. It's just really odd that you've come down with hay fever at this stage of your life. Can you tell me the symptoms you're getting?'

'Well, as soon as I step out of the house, my nose blocks up – immediately. And I can't breathe. So I simply turn tail and retreat back inside. That seems to do the trick.'

Lots of things about this feel puzzling. It's unusual to develop hay fever for the first time in your 70s. Also, I have never come across hay fever that is instantly cured by shutting the front door. And, come to think of it, it isn't just this conversation which is confusing me – there have been other times too when what he has said hasn't quite seemed to add up. It is like looking into a pool of water at a reflection which ever so briefly disintegrates before reassembling into a coherent image.

'The blocked nose sounds really annoying, but can you tell me a bit more about "weathering the storm"?'

There is a longish silence, enough to make me wonder if he hasn't understood what I mean or is annoyed that I have changed the subject.

'Well, it's all around isn't it, this virus? It's in the air everywhere. It could attack me at any time. And if it did attack, well of course that would be the end for me.'

'When was the last time you went out or saw anyone else?', I ask.

Another pause.

'100 days today, Dr. Shah. But you get used to it don't you?'

Do you get used to it? I wouldn't.

The rawness of his remark leaves me floundering, feeling ineffectual as I sit at my kitchen table. A small brown woman talking to an older, white man, from different social classes and different worlds. We feel very far apart just now and I think about how occupying the same space as someone else closes the distance in more ways than just the physical.

The conversation changes tack and becomes more practical again. I try to encourage him to take some short walks, to stop being afraid – of going out, of talking to people, of life, but I'm not sure if he really takes in what I say. I can't relieve him of his feeling that the outside world is a miasma of a deadly virus.

'And what about my hay fever?', he asks at the end of all this.

I think I will try to remember to call him again in a few days, before putting him out of my mind, logging back onto the computer system and calling the next patient on the list.

By the end of the surgery, I feel that my energy has ebbed away over the course of many such conversations. It's like eating fast food when you're hungry. The next day, I can only clearly recall patients I spoke to whom I already knew. The others have drifted away into an amorphous mass of names.

When the system is increasingly based on telephone triage medicine, physical and sensory shared experiences are removed. 'Assessment' is moved into a realm of numbers, scores, and escalation thresholds.

COVID-19 meant that face-to-face appointments had to be limited, in order to prevent the spread of the virus. Its advent accelerated a process of change that was already underway in general practice in the United Kingdom, as set out in the Long Term Plan. Some pioneering GP services had already adopted remote consulting, by telephone or video prior to Spring 2020. Online triage services were also gaining popularity – even before the pandemic, many surgeries required patients to fill in an electronic form describing their symptoms before they were offered an appointment. Mr. Sidwell's text messages were the result of a literal interpretation of what he put on this form. This type of triage relies on patients being reliable narrators of their illnesses.

In our surgery, the ratio of in-person:remote consulting used to be approximately 9:1 – this was reversed by the pandemic and although the ratio is drifting back, it seems unlikely that we will ever return entirely to the old way of doing things. The fact is that remote consulting is so much more convenient – for many patients and for GPs who for the first time have the option of working from home. Patients don't need to take time off work and to be kept waiting by over-stretched GPs, access is better for some people (although many GPs have been overwhelmed by the volume of online enquiries they receive and respond in a similarly transactional way – the double-edged sword of instant access).

Some of these changes in access are positive. But what risks being lost is connection. During remote consultations, although people assure me that it's convenient to talk, in reality they are busy – at a supermarket checkout counter, leaving their office desk to take calls in office bathrooms or in stairwells, running after kids in a park, having coffee with friends. And for the clinician, there are other distractions – imperfect technology, e-mails, blood results, and letters popping up on our screens which derail our attention.

As human beings, we use all our senses when we interact with people. For me (Rupal), touch has always been an important part of what I do. A handshake, holding someone's hand when they cry, feeling an abdomen, taking a pulse – all small, physical acts which form a connection. I miss the eye contact. Even though video consulting lets you see someone's face, we don't look in the same way or hold the gaze of the person we are speaking to. When someone is physically in the same room as me and I notice a change in tone or an averted gaze, I can use eye contact, a touch of the hand, and silence to help with the diagnosis and as part of the treatment. I don't understand how to interpret silence when the consultation is done virtually and I'm probably too quick to fill it. The small talk that is so natural when you see someone in person feels out of place somehow. Contact is more transactional, brisker, more medical, and less relational.

And communication through speech alone doesn't suit everybody. Sometimes physical gestures and facial expressions reveal more about meaning than words do. A system which relies on people being able to express themselves in order to access the right treatment is potentially discriminatory, and not only to those for whom English is a second language. Like Mr. Sidwell, even someone who is articulate in most circumstances might struggle to disclose something important that makes them vulnerable.

Patients have historically chosen who their GP will be based on whether or not there is a connection between them and the doctor they see. Many of my most important relationships with patients have been based on us liking each other, who can tell exactly why. It's hard to establish how much you like someone on the telephone when you haven't met. I can't see their face, they can't see mine. It's hard to get much deeper than a sympathetic chat. So, I wonder whether remote consulting is the nail in the coffin for continuity of care with one doctor – whether we will all become infinitely replaceable, more than we already are.

The Bad Mother

This is a fictional account of a consultation carried out remotely in the absence of any pre-existing relationship between doctor and patient.

Fifteen months after the birth of her son, Charlotte has days when she feels so numb that she questions whether she is still alive. She worries she is having a breakdown when the bad feelings that she can't control bubble and churn around inside her. She doesn't feel like herself anymore and wonders why the world feels so distant. It is like going through life wrapped up in a paper bag. She is so tired that sometimes she thinks that she could lock herself into her bedroom and sleep forever.

She loves William but finds it hard to engage with him and has been struggling even more now that he has started to have temper tantrums. She is too frightened to tell anyone that the last time this happened, she ended up leaving William in the flat on his own for ten minutes while she went out to clear her head – she thought at the time that she might hit him if she didn't. Although she has friends, these feelings are too shameful to voice to any of them and she is afraid of their judgement. She has been posting photos of herself and her husband with William on social media, which show the life she would like to have.

She has been a frequent attender at the surgery since William was born. She dreads seeing a GP in case they realize what an abysmal mother she is, but in her current state she is finding it impossible to trust her own judgement about whether or not it is safe to let an illness take its course, and so she needs to seek reassurance. She is worried when she receives a text from the surgery telling her that William won't be seen in person and that based on the information she submitted electronically to the surgery, she has been put on the list for a telephone call and that she should text back with photographs of William's rash.

It is a Monday morning, the telephone list is getting longer and the GP assigned to call Charlotte back hasn't ever met her before. She knows that the patient booked in after Charlotte is an elderly lady with multiple problems and is hoping that this will be a quick consultation to allow her to catch up. Charlotte's accent reveals her middle-class background and the GP experiences a stab of irritation at having to deal with another entitled, neurotic mother. She reads the blurb from the e-consult and wonders why Charlotte is unable to manage her son's minor illnesses herself.

During the telephone call, the GP doesn't see the pile of toys all over the floor, the unmade bed or the stain on Charlotte's blouse.

CHARLOTTE: William isn't well ... again. He isn't sleeping. And his eczema has flared up.

GP: Has he got a fever or cough? Is he short of breath?

CHARLOTTE: Erm ... no. I don't think so.

GP: That's good. Any other rash apart from eczema? Is he vomiting?

CHARLOTTE: No, but I don't think he's eating very well.

GP: Many children of William's age have eczema. And toddlers are often fussy about their food, don't worry. I've seen the photos you sent through and they're typical of eczema. You have the steroid cream on a repeat prescription. I think my colleague told you last time that you should just apply it for a few days during a flare up? You don't need to call in if it's not too severe. And don't forget to moisturise regularly.

CHARLOTTE: I didn't want him to have steroids ... isn't there an alternative?

GP *(exasperated)*: No, not really. Listen, a few days of a steroid cream is perfectly harmless, don't worry. Oh *(looking more carefully at the computer screen and alerts)* ... and don't forget to book for William's MMR – it's due now. It's really important to make sure you remember to get him vaccinated, so please make an appointment. You can do it via reception or online if you go to the practice's website. Ok, well I hope he gets better soon. Goodbye for now.

From the GP's point of view, there is nothing wrong with William. And she's right, she just hasn't understood that it is Charlotte and not William (yet) who needs help. At best, the consultation is a waste of time for everyone concerned and at worst, it is actively harmful. Unfortunately, that's never going to be captured in any audit of services. The health service is over-stretched, but trying to save time through quick, impersonal remote consultations can have the opposite effect. Patients and not the algorithm should determine whether their consultations are remote or in person. It should be part of the culture of medicine to exercise curiosity rather than judgement, even when the problem presented is seemingly trivial. Asking Charlotte a question like, 'What do you need?' might be important not only from a human, relational perspective, but also more cost effective in the long run.

No Decision about Me without Me

Despite NHS mission statements about care being centred around the patient, decisions are often made in multidisciplinary team meetings, which are attended by the different professionals involved in the care of the patient, but to which the patient is not invited. For example, a few times a year, we have a virtual meeting with one of the diabetes consultants from the local teaching hospital. A computer programme selects the patients most at risk of complications because their blood sugar control is poor. We then go through the list together – one of the GPs and the consultant – and the consultant suggests various changes to medications and referrals. He doesn't know any of the patients on the list and the GP will know only some of them. A collusion of anonymity.

The meetings generate a list of letters or calls to make to patients to explain why their drugs have changed or offering referral to the dietitian or the diabetic specialist nurse.

In some practices, GPs look through the computerized medical records of patients with diabetes and make management decisions on the basis of the numbers, which are then implemented by other staff such as healthcare assistants. It is a model which is becoming increasingly popular, not just for diabetes but for many other chronic conditions, despite the government's 2012 White Paper 'Liberating the NHS: No Decision about Me without Me'.

It is a bureaucratic approach, in which protocol and categorization are given the most power and in which decisions are made through the lens of the disease and not the patient, for the sake of efficiency.

But there are pitfalls and Yasmin's story is an example. The protocol advises that she should titrate up her dose of insulin and go to see a dietitian to discuss healthier eating strategies. Plus a referral to an exercise programme.

Yasmin is a 52-year-old interior designer who runs her own company. I have known her for about fifteen years now and have seen her quit her job, go back to university and then set up by herself. It hasn't been easy and has involved personal risk – if things hadn't worked out, there would have been no one to fall back on – she has never married and doesn't have a partner or children.

Outwardly, she is self-assured and successful. I'm sure it isn't obvious to those around her that her struggle with her weight, which has culminated with her developing type 2 diabetes has been a constant feature of her adult life. It's something that she has slowly divulged to me over many years. Even her closest friends don't know this about her.

She told me once that she was bullied at school for being fat. Her tone was light as she said it, passing it off as a casual remark, of no particular consequence. But I know that it is not inconsequential, that some things never quite leave you. I know what it was like to be an immigrant child in the 1970s – a shared understanding that we have never explicitly acknowledged to one another. She said she remembers the looks of disgust cast at her when she was eating her packed lunches as a child and the name-calling. This shame has never left her and she finds it hard to distance herself from the lonely, chubby schoolgirl who is her unwanted companion.

'I have always had to deal with being bigger than other people', she has said, and it is clear how much this matters, even though objectively, she is a fairly average size now. Although she is so successful at work, she spends hours each day worrying about what she will wear, how she looks, and what to choose to eat. She feels she is irredeemably ugly. She is engaged in a perpetual battle with food and she says she is disgusted with herself when she fails and gets up to binge eat at night when she can't sleep. She hates the insulin she is prescribed because it makes her gain weight and she would rather take a chance with the high sugars.

'You are an ugly, fat old woman. Why on earth would anyone ever love you?' The inner voice taunts her, so she continues to punish herself. One of my patients put it this way:

You know as you get older and flabbier, you need love more than when you are young. It's one of life's ironies that the sagging skin, the folds of fat, the new blemishes that keep appearing every year don't stop you from craving physical intimacy, needing to be held – they just mean it's less likely to happen.

When things get really bad, she self-medicates with alcohol and then feels guilty about the extra calories. She has had passing relationships, but nothing has ever stuck, nobody has managed to make her feel good about herself.

I have had many similar conversations with her over the years, and she has had repeated attempts at therapy. But the voice won't go away and so she continues to turn away opportunities in her personal life and refuse to believe that she is worth loving.

So when she gets a call after one of these virtual meetings suggesting a dietitian referral and an increase in her insulin dose, it is like a punch in the face. She loses faith in me. She trusted me and I should be able to protect her from harm. I am part of the practice, so actions from the team implicate me.

Galacticos – Out of Hours, Out of Time?

'Galacticos' is the ambiguous term used for the interstellar star ensemble of footballers signed up for the Real Madrid football team of the early 2000s. It stands for the collective of world-class players and also represents the policy of recruiting overpaid, ageing superstars. One young colleague mockingly referred to the group of seasoned GPs working in our local OoH service as 'Galacticos'.

But my colleagues JJ, Ben, and Dr. T are not overpaid Divas; they are hard-working generalists who can take on anything and everything at any time. In football terms or in the hierarchy of specialisms, they would be the substitutes who can play ANY position.

When I got stuck with a tricky question about palliative medicine on my first shift, I called Ben for advice. Ben is retired. The practice he retired from has a contract to cater for patients who have been expelled from other practices for bad behaviour. His clinical entries read like short novels written by a nineteenth-century great narrator. Period dramas. He did humanitarian work in Gaza. He has used his galactical OoH wages to build an arboretum. In one of his last shifts, he delivered a baby. He also attended my father-in-law when we had him living with us, to fulfil his wishes to die at home.

JJ is ageless and obviously fit. He runs marathons and probably will carry on doing so even after his death. In his last London Marathon, he fell but carried on and finished, in pain. The X-ray taken afterwards showed that he had broken his humerus. He carried on running and postponed the documentation of his injuries until after he finished the race.

Dr. T is the oldest Galactico. He must be in his 70s and during the first lockdown saw patients in all the local COVID-19-infested nursing homes; at the same time, some junior colleagues shielded themselves completely from any patient contact. He works long hours on weekends, he does Mental Health Act assessments, and one patient in the Mental Health Unit I look after remembers him as *his* GP in Penygroes, 'he is a legend'. Dr. T *is* a legend. He lost his driving licence because of drunk driving on a motorbike. He is the wounded healer. We fellow workmates wrote letters of support for him and he carries on. And on. And on. And on.

These doctors are living relics from the time of Dr. John Sassall, the Fortunate Man – the GP whose selfless service was documented by John Berger and who eventually committed suicide. They are fortunate, they are the Galacticos, and they are also slightly out of time.

In time, on point, are the remote assessments undertaken by low-trained, low-paid people operating the algorithm, the invisible Hogwarts sorting hat.

In the OoH service, our management system alongside the computer system has changed. Before June 2021, clinicians had access to all incoming calls and could select jobs local to their area. They had autonomy over their workload, which was grounded in their patch and they liked it.

The new system has cut them off from the incoming stream of calls. Everything is triaged by remote call handlers feeding the algorithm. Consequently, the workload has changed. There are more jobs triaged for ambulance and hospital admission, and the clinicians face more mundane tasks in the context of call centre medicine, which covers a much wider area now. Local knowledge is now irrelevant. The Galacticos may as well be sent to Pluto.

It leaves them frustrated. The absence of clinicians in other areas means that they must practise call centre medicine and allocate the finishing touches of a task to someone else. Nobody knows whether this 'someone else' is a real person, who is ready and waiting to see the patient, or whether they are a computer mirage. Often there are no appointments and the doctor on the phone is left managing an impossible task and impossible risk.

It makes me sad to see that lives of such rich lived experience have so little value. In the battle for autonomy and dominance, management alongside the opaque and dominant algorithm has won.

The power has shifted towards 'management' and algorithms. The Galacticos are on the way out, just at the time when their knowledge and skills are bitterly needed.

Reflection

Unintentional injustice can arise from systems which rely on patients being able to explain their symptoms accurately on an online form and to follow a flowchart of questions before being allowed access. It makes services more open to some than others, particularly where mental health is concerned. Remote consultations can disadvantage vulnerable patients who can't express what they are feeling, even if they don't come from materially disadvantaged backgrounds (see 'A Blocked Nose' and 'The Bad Mother' above). A systematic review concluded that remote consultations in general practice are likely to be used more by working people, non-immigrants, older patients, and women. It also concluded that internet-based consultations are more utilized by younger, affluent, and educated people.[13] There are currently no good quality analyses of the quality of remote consultations compared to in-person consultations and until there are, we should be careful about assuming there is no difference between them.

Poverty can lead to deepening inequalities in a system which relies on triage – poverty is associated with digital exclusion.[14] A report published in March 2022 found that 6 per cent of families in the United Kingdom do not have access to the internet and those most at risk of digital exclusion are the most financially vulnerable; those with hearing or vision impairment; and those who live alone.[15] Algorithms therefore inadvertently block access to health for the most disadvantaged groups in our society, leaving A&E the only viable option – a 2021 Red Cross report concluded that high-intensity A&E use is closely linked with wider inequalities and deprivation.[11] How do services accommodate the digital divide? Attrition and non-attendance are factors that have to be considered in the provision of services for users with high distress levels and chaotic lives.

Protocols and algorithms can never be used as a substitute for human judgement. Tate and Ahluwalia make a case for GP training which rewards the ability to notice and act on the particularities of the situation at hand.[16] Indeed, the healthcare system relies on its staff being able to take into account nuance and apply discretion when needed. Unfortunately, this is not the message that is received on the shop floor, and in our experience, healthcare staff are increasingly fearful of using their own judgement. Eliminating human beings from decision-making causes huge turbulence, inefficiency, and distress in a system which is already overburdened.

Notes

1. David Zigmond, 'The Perils of Industrialised Healthcare' (UK: Centre for Welfare Reform, 2019).

2. Kenneth V. Iserson and John C. Moskop, 'Triage in Medicine, Part I: Concept, History, and Types', *Annals of Emergency Medicine* 49, no. 3 (2007): 275–81.

3. Kaspar Villadsen and Ayo Wahlberg, 'The Government of Life: Managing Populations, Health and Scarcity', *Economy and Society* 44, no. 1 (2015): 1–17.

4. Rupal Shah and John Launer, 'Escaping the Scarcity Loop', *The Lancet* 394, no. 10193 (2019): 112–13.

5. Jacob A. Blythe and Farr A. Curlin, '"Just Do Your Job": Technology, Bureaucracy, and the Eclipse of Conscience in Contemporary Medicine', *Theoretical Medicine and Bioethics* 39, no. 6 (2018): 431–52.

6. Majority Staff of the Committee on Transportation and Infrastructure. 2020, https://www.edpierson.com/final-737-max-report-for-public-release.

7. 'NHS Long Term Plan', 2019, accessed December, 11, 2022, https://www.longtermplan.nhs.uk/.

8. Johanna Shapiro, 'Illness Narratives: Reliability, Authenticity and the Empathic Witness', *Medical Humanities*, vol. 37, no. 2, (2011): 68–72.

9. Eric J. Cassell, *The Nature of Healing: The Modern Practice of Medicine* (Oxford University Press, 2012).

10. Havi Carel, 'Phenomenology as a Resource for Patients', Paper Presented at the *Journal of Medicine and Philosophy: A Forum for Bioethics and Philosophy of Medicine*, 2012.

11. British Red Cross, *Nowhere Else to Turn: Exploring High Intensity Use of Accident and Emergency Services, A Summary Report 2021*, 2021.

12. Sara E. Shaw and Rebecca Rosen, 'Fragmentation: A Wicked Problem with an Integrated Solution?', *Journal of Health Services Research & Policy* 18, no. 1 (2013): 61–64.

13. Ruth F. Parker, Emma L. Figures, Charlotte A. M. Paddison, James I. D. M. Matheson, David N. Blane, and John A. Ford, 'Inequalities in General Practice Remote Consultations: A Systematic Review', *BJGP Open* 5, no. 3 (2021): BJGPO.2021.0040.

14. Anita Ramsetty and Cristin Adams, 'Impact of the Digital Divide in the Age of COVID-19', *Journal of the American Medical Informatics Association* 27, no. 7 (2020): 1147–48.

15. Ofcom, *Digital Exclusion: A Review of Ofcom's Research on Digital Exclusion Among Adults in the UK* (2022).

16. Andy Tate and Sanjiv Ahluwalia, 'A Pedagogy of the Particular – Towards Training Capable Gps', *Education for Primary Care* 30, no. 4 (2019): 198–201.

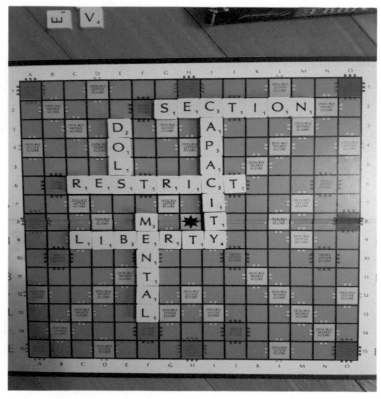

FIGURE 5.1: Scrabble 5, 'Freedom', Rupal Shah and Jens Foell, 2021.

5.
Taking Liberties: Regulating the Mental Health Act

Doctors' Roles in the Administration of Restriction of Civil Liberties

Doctors are agents of social control. Their expertise in health matters is used in the processes that can limit people's liberties. In the context of mental health, patients can be coerced into being assessed in secure units or receiving treatment against their will.

With some additional training, mainly around the interface of law, social work, and psychiatry, GPs can become approved assessors who participate in Mental Health Act (MHA) assessments (otherwise known as Section 12 assessments). They may be called upon if the police have picked up a confused person wandering in the street, or if people are behaving strangely or appear to be a risk to others or from others. Mental Health and social matters constitute a large proportion of police work. They jokingly call themselves 'social workers in uniform'. When welfare checks are carried out by the police, they are allowed to break people's doors down, in the pursuit of checking their health and confirming their whereabouts.

Interorganizational safeguarding meetings take place to provide a multifaceted perspective on the lives of people at risk. Occasionally, GPs take part in these meetings. Safeguarding conferences can also include representatives from the school, housing, police, probation, and legal services. What happens in the realm of healthcare is only one facet of a bigger picture.[1]

These meetings and processes regulate and embody power – the power to protect children and vulnerable adults. This includes the power to restrict civil liberties or to place people in care against their will.[2]

It is less well known that the liberties of people who lack the capacity to make decisions can also be restricted by 'DOLS' – the 'deprivation of liberty safeguards', which apply to supported living institutions in England and Wales.[3] They are informally known as the 'gilded cage', for which doctors are part of the legal framework holding the keys. The safeguards ensure that the door is locked, that there is a code at the door and that residents, often diagnosed with dementia, cannot escape their confined living environment.

The Puncture

The cast	
I (Jens)	Section 12 approved GP; father
Tracey	Approved Mental Health Professional (AMHP)
Dr. F	Psychiatrist
Daisy	The poodle
Mr. W	Intelligent patient diagnosed with dementia
Eva	Intelligent wife and caller for help
The Chorus	We: the Learners

On an occasional, ad hoc basis, I (Jens) am called to participate in MHA assessments. This process of social administration can – like legal punishments – strip people of their civil liberties and put them into confinement.

Being approved under Section 12 of the MHA requires training in understanding the shadowland between mental illness, psychiatry, the influences on mood, and the ability to make reasoned judgements. 'Insight' and the capacity to make decisions play a central role in this process. I put 'insight' into quotation marks because what exactly it means is often unclear to me, given its central role in the process of regulating confinement. An MHA assessment is serious business. The purpose of the assessment is to decide whether a person is detained under the MHA or not. It is a proper outcome-based business: at the end, there will either be a document or not. Either a pink form with text in black ink or none. Confinement or not.

The episode I am talking about highlights this dilemma.

It is Thursday morning. My day off. The phone rings. It is the AMHP covering Gwynedd. She says there is an 86-year-old man diagnosed with dementia, allegedly things are escalating, and they have received a distress call from his wife. The case has been handed over the previous day and she is not in possession of all the details. She gives me the name and address and we arrange to meet round the corner outside the house. The Psychiatrist will also attend.

We are meeting offsite in order not to stir up any apprehension. On the way to the property, we engage in a bit of small talk. Tracey moved to her current role because she was fed up of doing long shifts in social services Out-of-Hours. 'And you, where do YOU live?', I ask the Psychiatrist. 'In hospital accommodation', he says. He says that he got fed up with being tied down with his permanent job in Sussex and now works here on a locum basis. (A huge proportion of Gwynedd Mental Health Services is delivered by locum consultants.) He has seen Mr. W before. They informed me that Mr. W is/was a wealthy entrepreneur, allegedly he has properties in Italy and abroad. This is his second marriage and things are escalating. Apparently, his behaviour is erratic, though he is generally highly functioning. He has been diagnosed with dementia. We are walking on muddy streets in Gwynedd, an unexpected location for the mansion of a global player.

Act 1

Eventually, we find the house. It is not a mansion; it is an inconspicuous property with views of the marshes. We ring, the patient opens the door, and there is a bit of an awkward moment. Where shall we go? What shall we do? And how will we go about our mission? The wife is in the kitchen, and he is in the living room. No joint conversation. Without deciding on a timeframe and strategy we start operating separately. It is not really a planned decision. The Psychiatrist and Social Worker are heading to the kitchen, the main stage, to speak with the wife (the caller-for-help), so I think I'll stay offstage with the patient whilst they make significant enquiries.

The patient is sitting on the couch. Daisy the poodle is sitting next to him and is being cuddled by him throughout the conversation. He speaks calmly about being diagnosed with dementia and that he knew something was not right with him, but he is functioning. He gets dressed and goes for walks. He is insightful about his predicament though I notice that at times he grasps for words during the interview. After a bit of hesitancy, the words come, not always with utmost precision, but the interview has a coherent flow.

He comes from Italy, so I mobilize my rudimentary Italian conversational skills to establish a connection. They are good enough to find out where he is from, how long he has been here in the United Kingdom, etc. He tells me that he was raised in Emilia Romagna but moved to Rome. That his mother Filomena was brought up by the clergy because her parents were too poor to raise her. That he loves her. That she was an intelligent woman. And that he is an intelligent man. Being intelligent has provided many opportunities in his life. He excelled in school and became an engineer. He worked for Ferrari in Italy and later in Germany, and then he moved to the United Kingdom. Here, he worked for McLaren, he had his peak in the booming car industry of the 1960s and 1970s. He operated worldwide. He met his first wife in London. She is from Wales; they moved back to North Wales. He does not have UK citizenship, because he is not British, he is Italian.

(Snap! I feel the same. I am German, I live here, and my life is here, but I am German. I am not British. He seems to have made similar choices regarding belonging.)

He tells me that he has sold his Italian properties and there is not much left for him in Italy. He will not return. He has lived his life in the United Kingdom and will stay here.

(Maybe the same will apply to me later after retirement? The Immigrant's dilemma?)

He tells me that his first marriage ended in divorce. That he had an active working life all over the world, and at one time his wife said that it was not working for her, so they divorced, he said, and he supported her in finding a new place to live. He is in contact with her, but they don't see each other anymore. He also has contact with his four children from his first marriage but does not see them either. In his current marriage, he sees similar developments developing.

(Snap! I have an active, intellectually and financially rewarding life with opportunities, but work commitments and family commitments are often difficult to reconcile.)

After the divorce, he met his current wife, Eva. 'An intelligent woman.'

(On a dating platform? Arranged second marriage? I cannot work out the photos on the walls. I am guessing they have no biological children of their own, and the children are from their first relationships.)

The flow takes us to the role of the Catholic Church in Italy (his mother Filomena was raised by nuns but opted out aged 18 and had him). He resents the Church. Subsequent topics in the flow of conversation are life in London in the 1960s. His stories make me think of the swinging 60s, Bar Italia, Soho, the role of sex, and free love.

There is a pause. It does not feel like a meaningful pause and I do not suspect what comes next.

He makes a sign with his hands, indicating about 7 cm between his thumb and index finger. He says that this is his size. That's all he has. And that his wife wanted a lot of sex. That it used to bother him, but now he accepts the size of his penis.

(I do not know what to say. Does size matter? Whose problem is it? Is this HIS problem or something his wife complained about and demanded? He had four children. Something must have worked. 'It is not the size of the waves; it is the motion of the ocean', they say, [...] but how can I bring this into the conversation; [...] should I bring this into the conversation? Our offstage lounge conversation gets to the core issues of male pride: intelligence, being able to provide and satisfy, and penis size.)

We speak about cars. His life with engines and cars. He says that Dr. F injured him badly by stripping him of his licence to drive. That it was wrong, despite the diagnosis of dementia he could always drive. Losing this affected him badly.

He says that yesterday he went out to the car and punched it. He does not remember what exactly triggered it, but he regrets it and won't do it again.

He says that in the past he became angry quickly, but this has always been a verbal mood eruption, that he is a gentleman, he would never become violent, and had never become violent.

We talk about his current relationship with Eva. He knows she wants to end the relationship. What next? He speaks about supported living, 'a hospital', all rather vague.

(How is the threshold between verbal aggression, aggression against inanimate objects and against other bodies, and other people configured? What triggers transgressions? It makes me think of my daughter. Her mood is certainly volatile. Objects fly, doors get slammed, and verbal assaults are deployed with massive impact. What configures the borderline between mood management with our nearest and dearest and a civil code of conduct? When is this a case for the police, social workers or healthcare workers? I would like to ask under what circumstances he may or will become violent again, what are the triggers, and when does he flip? I missed the opportunity to ask these questions.)

Act 2

Dr. F and Tracey are moving from the kitchen into the lounge. Mr. W is sitting on the sofa. Daisy is heading towards Dr. F to sniff him out. He moves back and asks Mr. W to remove Daisy. The conversation now has a more normative flavour. It is about the reason Eva called us and what led up to this escalation. Eva called because Mr. W attacked the car with a knife and punctured three tyres. She also mentioned verbal threats. She said she does not feel safe anymore. This had been established by Dr. F and Tracey in the kitchen, whilst Mr. W and I were chatting in the living room.

Now the three of us are convening in the living room for the more normative part of the conversation. Mr. W is accused of having stuck his knife into the tyres of his/their car.

This is not just any object. This is the car. His car. The car he is not allowed to drive any more. The car his wife could use to get away from him. The wife who is about to end her relationship with him. He spent his life in the car industry. He is a motor engineer.

Mr. W starts this round by clearing the air with Dr. F. 'You know you hurt me badly when you took my licence away.' Dr. F is taken aback by this. It takes some moments for him to connect with what Mr. W is alluding to.

Dr. F moves to a combination of bureaucratic speak ('It is part of *our* obligation to inform the DVLA.') and expression of understanding Mr. W's frustration. Mr. W had been referred to have a driving test, and unfortunately, he failed this test. He says that the instructor made a mistake and gave misleading instructions or comments on a roundabout and this led to him having to hand his driving licence in.

He says this has been a massive blow for him, but he accepts it, just as he accepts his diagnosis.

We are talking about anger.

'Your affect is labile', says Dr. F. He offers low-dose antipsychotics to help equilibrate the fluctuating mood.

Mr. W reiterates that he is a gentleman, he would never be violent, and he accepts his diagnosis and the limitations it brings to his life.

Dr. F states that his act of violence is seen in the framework of domestic violence; it will be reported to the police and if it happens again, he is likely to be sectioned. His voice is calm when he says this, Mr. W is also calm. The narrative-normative flow is now less turbulent.

We are talking about life and lifestyle. Mr. W says that he looks after himself, goes for regular walks, and has a strong body. At the same time, he says that he feels that something is not right in his body and he will die soon. He just says it.

This utterance triggers a set of questions by Dr. F. 'How are you sleeping? How is your appetite?', the routine set of questions regarding depression is to follow. The answer is No, No, No. All normal.

Conversations can be a dance, can be a fight. Bruce Lee speaks about Wu-Wei, non-doing. How would a Taoist approach to such conversations look? The agenda-led outcome-based process of conversations in the context of an MHA assessment moves us clearly to an outcome: Mr. W is not detainable under the MHA. His anger is an issue, and this will be followed up by police and mental health services under the label 'anger management'. Labelled with 'affect lability', he will be treated with low-dose antipsychotics which should act as mood stabilizers. It is strongly recommended that he and his wife seek professional support in dealing with their relationship issues.

I advise Mr. W to 'get his house in order' – finances, care arrangements, advance directives. Time is ticking for him.

This phase of the conversation is very advice-and-decision-heavy. Clearly on the normative side.

Act 3

The drama goes into the third round: the three agents of social control move to the kitchen to relay the verdict to Eva, the caller.

On the shelf is a bottle of Barolo. I have seen it at Lidl, £11 per bottle. Mr. W said earlier that he used to drink heavily in the past. Now a glass with food. No more. Maybe one and a half. And that Eva detests wine. She won't have any. She hates alcohol.

The door to the living room is half open. Mr. W sits in the living room, and his wife sits at the kitchen table. Nothing is going on between them, no verbal negotiation, no small talk. Daisy does not know where to go. And she has to cope with the intruders in the kitchen space. Dr. F shoos her away again.

We tell Eva that rather than sending Mr. W into confinement, we have decided to offer a range of support in the community. 'He does not meet the requirements for being sectioned.'

The domestic violence unit at the police force will be involved. This will also open some doors for support, including anger management for Mr. W. We strongly suggest seeking help in the matter of their relationship, counselling or reconciliation. We suggest Mr. W has support in managing his financial matters.

This is not what Eva wanted to hear. She wanted him to be locked up. 'He needs HELP', she says, insinuating that HELP will be available on the ward and that what she is being offered now is not the HELP she expected when she made the call.

(She does not say 'I need help'. What difference would it make if she put herself in the centre? If it was not about him, if it was about her?

She does not know that the dementia ward serves a different clientele. Whenever I visit this ward, I see people holding dolls, shouting and screaming people, people who are in the end stages of dementia or displaying very disruptive behaviour.)

Eva invites us to look back into his biography rather than focusing on current biology. 'Did you ask his children why they are not talking to him?' But this is not the topic of this encounter. Eva exudes discontent, even passive aggression at the outcome.

Epilogue

We are leaving the house as a group and are walking to our cars to get on with our daily lives. Technically, this joint assessment is a combination of timely and spatially layered sub-conversations. If it had been a therapeutic event, I would have liked to ask questions like 'What would happen if nothing happens?', 'What is the best that could happen?' I would have liked to ask Mr. W how he is dealing with this decline in influence, control, and life radius in view of his past achievements.

A crime forecaster at the police once told me that they can predict domestic violence, 'males become violent when their partner ends the relationship'. Exactly this happened with Mr. W and at exactly this point in time he attacked the car, her getaway vehicle. Unexplained? Incomprehensible? Will never happen again?

I felt the palpable discrepancy between her perspective and his and wondered how they can carry on living under one roof. As much as it was clear that detaining Mr. W under the framework of the MHA would have been a misjudgement, I wondered what other options they had, realistically.

I contacted Mr. W's surgery to convey to them his idea that he feels something is wrong in his body. I was mindful of the two ways he portrayed his body as both resilient ('I walk the dog every day ... I am strong.') yet simultaneously decaying ('I know there is something wrong ... I feel it ... I will die soon.'). I kept asking myself why he was so accepting and so insightful. Had he given up? Was the attack on the car the last act of the ageing, raging male facing his final decline?

Did we as a group of professionals have more power than we thought and could we have used the unusual synergy of Consultant Psychiatrist, Social Worker, and GP as a therapeutic event?

I met Tracey afterwards in a separate, unrelated event. She said that Mr. W had a history of controlling behaviour, ripping credit cards up, etc. That this is an ongoing and evolving situation.

In the book *Rapport*, psychologists Emily and Laurence Alison talk about their work with investigative and legislative dialogues in the police force.[4] According to them, the good cop is the better cop. They categorize four prototypes of dialogue styles: T-Rex (confrontation), Mouse (capitulation), Lion (control), and Monkey (cooperation). And even in the context of incarceration, techniques inviting rapport are more successful than others. Similarly, successful interviewers challenge inconsistencies in narratives with curiosity rather than judgement. I could have done more of this in my conversation with Mr. W – 'Tell me more about your body as a resilient body versus your body as a vulnerable body'. Or: 'Under what circumstances will you become angry or lose your temper?', 'How does the prospect of losing yet another relationship in times of inevitable loss and frailty affect you as a man?'

Control is obviously the key in this mini-drama. This also applies to conversational strategies used when deciding the administrative endpoint in such situations: to section or not to section. I am realizing how many overt and covert conversations and relationships are interwoven in the fabric of this story.

A Supernatural Demonic Attack

When is it appropriate to detain people against their will? Is this a question of whether somebody has a 'disorder of the mind' or is it a question of the timely availability of support systems?

The story seemed to be clear-cut. The Social Worker told me that a disturbed woman had been picked up by the police. She was 'behaving strangely' and appeared to be distressed. Allegedly she was agitated, shouted utterances with religious content and was very difficult to deal with during her journey to the place of safety, a room in the local Accident and Emergency (A&E) Department. She had been taken to A&E, where they struggled with her. Then she was then transferred to the Mental Health Unit and had another dose of haloperidol and lorazepam, medications to calm her down.

The nurse in charge introduced the patient to me as being agitated and difficult to control.

She was in the '136 suite', a bare, locked room with windows, a bathroom, a wipeable sofa, and wipeable chairs. A rage-proof room with CCTV. We could see on the screen that the patient was pacing up and down. 'We' consisted of the nurse in charge, the approved mental health professional 'AMPH' (Social Worker), her colleague in training, and me.

I introduced myself and conscientiously asked short questions that followed the thread of the patients' narrative. Going with this flow, her narrative took us listeners to her spiritual orientation and her spiritual congregation. She spoke about her dog and the increasing distress that voices disguised as spirits caused her. She called this a 'supernatural demonic attack', and it led her to leave her house in distress. I had to interject with some medical questions but introduced them as such. The purpose of this interview was to determine whether she should be detained against her will under the MHA Section 2, or whether there were other, less restrictive options. It was 8 pm and no other services were available.

In contrast to what I had been told, and in contrast to the psychiatrist's recommendation, I thought that there was no reason to detain her under the MHA.

But then what?

'I am going now.'

'No, you can't, you are detained under Section 136 and for up to 24 hours, you are not a free citizen.'

I found it difficult. Yes, here, and now, under the influence of heavily pacifying medicines she was calm and collected. But how long would this last? Longer than the half-life of the medication she had been given? And then back to square one, back in the loop?

'Yes', she said, she has experienced a supernatural demonic attack, and this was distressing, and she was distressed, but is this a reason for treatment and observation in a locked environment against her will? What is the risk to herself? What is the risk to others? But what is the risk *from* others, if she, a vulnerable, disturbed person, is allowed to act strangely, shouting 'Jesus' on a street in North Wales? And would the same apply to a street in London? What is the wisest decision?

It took a long time.

She said, 'I am going home now'. We called family members. Like in *Who Wants to Be a Millionaire?*, she suggested we ask a friend, and she would stay with the friend. But could this member of the congregation be burdened or trusted with looking after a patient with acute, florid psychosis?

It boiled down to trust.

'Do you not trust me?'

'Yes, I do.'

'Then, can I go now?'

'What if you experience supernatural demonic attacks again and the police pick you up?'

I said I trusted her, but that didn't satisfy my need for control. And that she must stay overnight to give the system time to get hold of her community services, home treatment team, etc.

It felt like not allowing my daughter to go out to town on a Saturday evening.

I decided that more time was needed. That I could not decide at this point of the night. That I would play on time, like a football team when the purpose of the game is simply to play the game down the clock.

'You are very thorough', said the Social Worker in an ambiguous tone.

The next day, on my return, everything eventually turned out to be ok. The care coordinator said she would get in contact with the patient again. She could go home. She was NOT detained. I went against the psychiatrist's recommendation.

The majority of this decision-making depended on having a fluent and flowing conversation and believing what she said. This was not *non*-violent. Because she was already detained under Section 136, which lasts for 24 hours, I had the power to decide whether or not to detain her for longer by placing her under section 2 (this lasts for up to 28 days). I used it to buy time to get the system in gear – I used the structural violence and asymmetry of the relationship. However, it can be seen as an example of going the extra mile. In this instance, it consisted of spending two hours with her in the evening and returning the next day.

What I haven't written about is how I perceived her. With her Christian beliefs, her reciting of the Bible, and also what she told me about her childhood, I felt for her. I thought she would not benefit from being locked up. What is the point of locking up misfits?

I learned later that she started feeling better and subsequently stopped taking the medication, that she stopped communicating with the care coordinator and slowly became increasingly disturbed, like Travis in the film *Taxi Driver*, with the significant difference that for her, it did not result in acts of violence. It resulted in shouting religious utterances in public.

Tatort
Control and Relational Violence

There is a German TV institution: *Tatort*. Each Sunday evening at prime time, a crime thriller is broadcast. It is a federal product, so each region can proudly spotlight their unique geography as the backdrop for a crime plot. There is a commonly occurring final scene, much more common in German TV crime novels than in UK novels – the back of an ambulance is shown as an alternative to death.

Exactly this happened when I did a night shift.

When I arrived at work, my heart sank: there were already fifteen visits on the screen. Fifteen visits between Tywyn and Bodorgan. Impossible! The blurb for the one coded as 'urgent' was very extensive, but I thought I had better call first anyway, to get my own impression and prepare the essentials. The blurb mentioned that the call came from the husband of a woman whose behaviour had become problematic. A mental health problem. Allegedly she had previously experienced puerperal psychosis and intermittent psychotic episodes in the past but had been calm for the last few years.

I phoned, she answered. She asked when I would arrive and carried on, saying that I would need to section her husband, as he was the problem. He would need to go to a secure unit. She told me that he was controlling, he was a control freak. She said she had had enough of it now, she just needed to sleep.

I tried small talk, wanted to connect, but it did not work. I asked her where does she live? What does she do? She answered, 'Haven't you read the description I have already given?' Everything was aggression, ranging from passive to active aggression.

Back at the base, I felt this call needed preparation. I called the mental health unit – yes, she was known to their services but was now discharged back into the community. 'If there is a problem, send her to A&E and Psych liaison will deal with her.' Section her? Also, a possibility, but setting this up is a slow and bureaucratic process. Or the police – if there are safety issues, the police can intervene. If the behaviour occurs in the public realm, which means outside the home, a Section 136 can be applied. I spoke to the Consultant, and as expected he had a very distant attitude. He knew that many other people could be interjected between the trouble and him – GPs, mental health nurses, paramedics, police staff, emergency staff, community mental health workers, etc.

The scene was a grey, pebble-dash bungalow in a village full of other, similar rural dwellings. One could see the shadows of people pacing up and down like characters in an Indonesian shadow puppet theatre. A skip was located in the front garden, piled high with domestic bric-a-brac, including toys and children's clothes.

On entering the scene, I was immediately sucked into the drama. 'You have to calm her down', shouted the husband.

'Get out of here, get out', she yelled back. 'All of you get out, f*** off all of you, you can all f*** right off.'

The protagonists were a woman in her late 30s, dressed in a fluffy nightgown, her husband, dressed casually, looking concerned and calm, and his father, a man in his 70s, looking scared. No child. The child had been removed from the scene and was staying with his grandmother. I could not talk to the wife. Nothing would register with her. She was on a rampage. Pure rage. Language like in a pub, late on a boozy night out.

'F***, F*** F*** MONG F*** RETARD F*** F***.'

She pushed me out of the house. The husband urged me to solve the situation.

'Can you not give her lorazepam? That helped in the past!', he suggested.

I felt that he wanted to be the animal doctor in a wildlife programme, ready to blow a ketamine dart to de-escalate the situation. But this option was not an option, and I didn't have lorazepam with me. He said, 'It can't go on like this'.

I said, 'What if it does?'

'It can't.'

'What then?'

I told him we could call an ambulance, take her to A&E, and that we could take things from there.

'She will never agree.'

Or we could call the police, this is a situation of escalating domestic violence.

'I am a policeman, that would be very difficult, my colleagues would come and find out what's going on here.'

I said, 'I understand, but those are the options. Or we could organise the home treatment team, but that will take time to set up and certainly not materialize before Monday morning.'

I went back to the car to call the psychiatrist and write my report. I was still in sight of the Javanese puppet theatre. And the movements of the shadow puppets got faster, the situation was escalating. The father-in-law ran out and said to me, 'You need to call the police, she is hitting out.'

I called the police. I called Psychiatry.

Still a stand-off: they are in a domestic environment. If the police intervene, they will do so by exercising their power to protect others, so the wife will be subject to prosecution.

With matters as they are now, it was still unclear where she would end up. If the police intervened at home, her destination would be a police cell, not a mental health unit or A&E. If she left her house and entered the public sphere, she could be sectioned, but this wasn't possible on her private territory.

The police arrived. Understandably, they were not keen on getting involved in a messy situation, especially since she was not armed (the kitchen knives had been removed by her husband). They asked questions: 'Does she have capacity?'

Capacity to reflect on the question of whether it is appropriate to go to hospital, what the consequences are of not going, to be able to weigh up the pros and cons, and to retain this information. Difficult to say. She was on a rampage; I could not engage with her, and she did not remember what time it was (but she had different priorities!). It was like asking if a drunk person has capacity, whose conversation is stuck in a loop and whose emotional and intellectual flexibility has gone (for the moment, but sometimes this moment lasts a bit longer).

The police seemed not to be the right set of people to get her treatment, only the right set of people to get her out of the house. Once she was out, I called an ambulance. A telephone conversation with emergency services is a very rigid procedure. And resources are scarce. The section about 'threat to life' defines in which waiting bracket people are placed. I said this wasn't an immediate threat to life, but something needed to happen sooner rather than later. It was an escalating, unfolding mental health situation.

There were more figures in the Javanese puppet theatre. Movements. Hectic gesticulation. Then two police people escorted her out. She was handcuffed. She was placed in the back of the police van, behind the grid.

Then the policewoman ran to me and yelled, 'She is fitting, she is fitting!'

Indeed, she was lying on the floor, body jerking, blood-stained froth coming from her mouth, teeth grinding, skin purple. I ran back to the car and got the oxygen and the rectal diazepam to stop the fit.

A paradigm change: the situation now was a medical situation. She was a patient and not a prisoner. I had access to her body, her husband held her head, and the father-in-law got a blanket from the house. We could talk. She had calmed down. She was cold. She was lying in the back of a police van as we waited for the ambulance. I called back to upgrade the job to 'immediate threat to life'. The response to this immediate threat to life still took 45 minutes; 45 minutes of holding, measuring, and talking.

The husband said, 'She can't deal with stress. [...] We are renovating the house and preparing for the arrival of a puppy dog, a chocolate Labrador. And we have building work, which takes ages, nothing is working here, the builders just don't turn up, she can't cope with the stress'. He said that in the past there had been crisis episodes, but that recently, things had been stable. Finally, the ambulance came.

This would have been the final scene in the German *Tatort*: the protagonist sits on a stretcher. Emergency workers in uniform apply the medical paraphernalia, and the backdoor closes. End of the episode. I went back to our car. On leaving, the paramedics waved to me from the cockpit of their van, and I waved back from the passenger seat of the Skoda Scout with 'Meddyg' written on the roof.

The night went on.

The next day I enquired about her whereabouts in the local hospital. I learned that she was still in A&E, so I visited her in the bay. She greeted me with a friendly smile, said 'Thank you', and apologized for having thrown me out of her house. She said she was feeling ok now. She said that she had been very, very angry. That her husband does not follow instructions. Her instructions. That she is working from home and nothing has been working out. That he never listens.

I said that following rules, making rules, and controlling are big themes and that dysfunction is common.

She had several investigations because this was the first time she had had a seizure. There were brain changes on a CT scan. Inflammation of the brain? What was this? The power of emotions, an emotional drama culminating in a seizure. Brain inflammation immersed in the ingredients of the individual lifeworld? A recurring mental health problem, 'she can't cope with stress'?

Or is it a mixture of all and the weighting of the individual components is in the eye of the beholder?

Who has control? What are the boundaries for relational violence? What does it take to regain control?

I Am Dead

'I am dead', said the 17 years, 11-month-old child/adolescent/young woman to me during an MHA assessment.

We were in a quiet room in A&E. This is where difficult conversations are placed, where bad news is discussed. It is a place without technical paraphernalia, the place for psychosocial matters in emergency departments.

This was indeed a psychosocial matter. Eve had been brought in after attempts to harm herself. The CAMHS Psychiatrist had recommended that Eve should be admitted under Section 2 of the MHA – this would result in her being locked up for a period of assessment.

My role was to endorse or reject this decision.

There are two aspects to this process. One is whether this is in principle the right thing to do, whether she has a mental disorder that needs assessment, and the other aspect is what the alternatives could be. It is a Saturday evening; she is stranded in A&E and she is nearly 18.

Where could she go? What place is equipped to deal with her?

I heard that she cut herself, barricaded herself in the toilet, tried to escape, and is at high risk of 'death by misadventure'. I read in the notes that she had jumped off bridges in the past and had tried all sorts of harmful acts to injure herself. The notes mentioned complex post-traumatic stress disorder, I heard about plans to engage her in trauma therapy, about 'Eye movement desensitization and reprocessing', a psychophysiological procedure to reset troublesome memories. I read that her parents have no parental responsibility; this responsibility has been transferred to the local authorities. The Council are her parents. Panels of professionals decide her pocket money, her freedom to go out at night, and her future. I read she wants to pursue a career in childcare.

It is alleged that she was sexually attacked in the very space that was designed to protect her. Police got involved, and she was moved to an emergency placement in a house in Anglesey, supported/supervised by two people all the time. Their job is to prevent her from harming herself, from taking her life, or from sustaining avoidable injuries.

I read that apparently her emotional processing skills are low and that she meets the criteria for autism spectrum disorder and attention deficit hyperactivity disorder. I read that she is deemed to be at risk of 'CSE', childhood sexual exploitation. That's what happened. That's why she is here now, in the Emergency Department in the quiet room.

After having read the notes and being briefed by the Social Worker, I walked down the corridor of the Emergency Department. It looks like the busy environment one sees portrayed in medical TV dramas. Professionals with tunnel vision in different colour-coded uniforms that signify their rank in the hierarchy are rushing down the long corridor.

Two people in high-viz uniforms are placed in front of a door. They resemble policemen, but they are not, their uniform is not black. One guy is a colossus with tattoos and a long biker beard. There is no way of escape if he places himself in front of the door. They are protecting Eve from escaping, which is what she usually does.

On entering the room, I see Eve seated on a sofa. There is an adult standing next to her, from the Council (technically representing the parent role) who says she does not know her. Also, a woman is dressed in green, which marks her out as a Healthcare Assistant.

There is not much talk, nor much drama. I introduce myself and the purpose of this encounter. Eve must be bored of this. She has been sectioned on numerous occasions. On asking what she expects to happen, she replies that she expects to be placed in adult care. The thought of her being admitted to an adult psychiatric ward in a secure environment is awful, but so is the thought of her being in a paediatric ward next to children with middle ear infections, croup, diarrhoea, or other medical childhood predicaments.

Next to Eve is an unopened dream catcher.

'Where is this dream catcher from?'

'From my father.'

'How did you get it?'

'He sent it by post.'

He apparently lives in the next village. Why does he send it by post?

I understand Eve is estranged from her family and assume that bad things must have happened in her family. But bad things have also happened in the environment designed to protect her.

She is about to move from paediatric services to adult services. This means that a lot of support will be removed from her. She is very likely to fall into the gap between child and adult services, just when she needs the most support.

I ask all sorts of questions about what makes her tick, what music she likes, what food she likes, how she sleeps, and whether she has pets. Yes, she has two hamsters, she brought them from her placement in South Wales, the one that ended with police investigations and emergency resettlement. And now this emergency resettlement has also broken down due to the inability of her custodians to stop her from harming herself.

She has nowhere to go.

I ask where she thinks she would be safe. 'Nowhere', she says. I think she is right.

'I am not here', she says.

'Where are you then?', I reply.

'I am dead', she says.

And that's how it looks. No eye contact, no hope, and nowhere to go, I feel she has retreated into her mind, her emotions are in a place no one has access to, possibly not even herself.

I say that I would like to ask so many more questions, but not here and now, not in this environment. This is not about building trust. She knows this is a MHA assessment, she knows the score. She has been here before. I say that in view of her intentions to hurt herself and end her life, I have to place her on a section in a secure environment. This is easier said than done because at this point in time there are no such places, no 'beds' at all for her in North Wales.

She doesn't respond. She is in her dissociated space and has left her body as an empty shell behind.

In a side room, I write my version of the story and why I support the Psychiatrist's recommendation to place her in a secure environment. It is a pink form and the people who read it will pick up on the formalities, whether her address is accurate in all details. But I have never ever had anyone comment on my text. The bureaucratic regulation is geared towards the letter of the law, not the spirit. I find this bizarre – that no one has ever asked about my free text, but that on plenty of occasions, I have had to redo the formalities of the address.

Signing the pink document makes me very sad. I am thinking about 'insight' – and how the lack of it is a sign of a mental health disorder.

She said that nowhere is safe. That she is dead. In a biographical sense this is true, I think.

On leaving the department, I see that she tried again to escape. The colossus placed himself in front of the exit door of the department and she battled against him.

We are all trapped in a loop with no escape, it seems.

Double Agents - The Soap Operas and Tragicomedies of Primary Care

Doctors are not autonomous. They are governed by the GMC. Their licence to practise gets renewed every five years. They are obliged to engage in a yearly review of their professional performance, called appraisal, usually conducted by a colleague from the same profession, but (in order to avoid collusion) not from the same department or practice. In this appraisal of their professional learning, doctors must record complaints and significant events. They are also encouraged to reflect on difficult and ambiguous episodes of clinical care. The colleagues who review these logbooks of learning (appraisers) report back to the GMC, and thus occupy the role of a double agent. On the one hand, they represent the GMC and the population at large and must protect patients from bad practice. They are tasked with finding the bad apples and removing them or preventing them from getting worse. On the other hand, appraisals can provide a safe space for (appraisee) doctors to think about what they are doing, what is holding them back, what is going right, and what is going wrong. Appraisals oscillate between career counselling, life coaching, and the dynamics of control or even an investigation. Appraisers are double agents with dual commitments. I (Jens) am one of them. As an appraiser I am a double agent because I act as an agent of control. I am paid by National Health Service England and report to the Appraisal Lead, within a hierarchy of governance. I am not employed as a career coach, but often I act as one.

This double agency is well-trodden ground for street-level bureaucrats not only from general practice but also from different professions, including teachers and social workers and probation workers. Part of our remit is to act as agents of social control, and our salaries come from organizations and not from the individuals we monitor.

From time to time, I carry out appraisals (and, of course, I get appraised myself). Appraisals provide an opportunity to peek into others' work lives, snoop in other workplaces, and learn from others' mistakes and successes.

Reflections on difficult clinical cases included in appraisals often read like soap operas or dramatic novels, with twists and sudden turns. The lives of families with multi-generational experiences of abuse and violence are a GP's daily bread and

145

butter. Any GP with deep roots in their locality knows the family trees of families where trouble follows trouble. If children or vulnerable adults are harmed or at risk of harm, social services can put safeguarding measures into place. These measures vary in severity and range from giving extra support to struggling families – to forcibly placing the people who are cared for into a different environment under the supervision of social services.

GPs are legally obliged to share data and participate in safeguarding procedures. The emotional intensity of this participation varies from sharing data about someone not known to the practice, all the way through to painful disclosures involving people about whom the GP has intimate knowledge based on long-standing relationships – people who have been hurt and people who hurt others. In this way, the role of the GP mimics my role as an appraiser/double agent. Dual commitments. The quality of our work relies on the trustworthiness of the relationship, but exceptions to confidentiality and a degree of double-crossing are built into the contract.

Leslie's Story

I am appraising Leslie and reading her reflections about a case concerning Ms. N. Leslie is Ms. N's GP and, as such, is her advocate. She knows Ms. N and her two sons well. She has had to write numerous letters about the sons over the years. They have rarely been in school – Ms. N states this is because they have chronic fatigue syndrome. But they are missing out on life. Ms. N is also a patient in the practice but now avoids Leslie after she found out that Leslie had arranged a professionals' meeting, an event 'about you, without you'. For Ms. N this was an act of double-crossing and trust faded from the relationship. However, that is not the end of the story. There are ongoing suspicions that this could be a case of 'fabricated illness', that Ms. N has actively deceived doctors and nurses and pretended that her children are more ill than they really are. Leslie is still involved. She writes letters to new Consultants and new Social Workers. The story goes on. And on. And on.

The only way to support the sons is through a trusted relationship, but exactly this is hampered by the process of control and surveillance. Leslie is walking a tightrope. She must mince every word in the statements she makes. As an appraiser I can see the sediments of such entrenched and long-standing dramas as ongoing extended case reviews. No GP trainee will ever get tested on how they calibrate their loyalties over time, on the impact such a relationship may have on others in the practice, how practice politics inform their involvement in the case, and how what happens in people's personal lives spills over into professional commitments (and vice versa). Maybe it isn't so different from a TV drama, where the private lives of the protagonists are enmeshed and entangled with the plot of the episode.

Toni's Story

Toni, another appraisee, looks after three generations of the P's. In their country of origin, the P's were oppressed and marginalized. Things are not improving for them in the United Kingdom. There are safeguarding measures in place for the newest family member, Baby C. C's mother fought very hard to conceive. Everything in her life has been dramatic. Relationships have been volatile, and the relationships within the P family tree are no less volatile. The baby has been placed in foster care after the grandmother who holds the strings in the family allegedly dropped him. How likely is it that this was unintentional? BUT the grandmother has multiple medical conditions and chronic pain. She is on high doses of numbing painkillers. Toni must navigate her role as supporting the grandmother, the daughter, and the whole fragile and contradictory conflict-rich family.

Stories like this are often told by GPs to one another but are rarely documented with genograms and lines of relationships in the electronic patient record. The health record is individualized and belongs to the Health Authority. GPs can only curate it. But the story of general practice is made up of interdependent stories across the boundaries between patients and professionals. This mycelium of connected systems of relationships influences communities – for better or worse. I, Jens, street-level bureaucrat, double agent, observe this interconnectedness through the lens of significant event reviews, case reviews, learning logs, complaints, and compliments in the appraisals of other street-level bureaucrats and double agents with dual accountabilities.

Reflection

Thomas Hobbes wrote his book *The Leviathan* after the English civil war.[5] It features the regulation of passions in a civil society. Doctors play a huge role in the governance and regulation of passions, emotions, and sanity in our society. Doctors are given the task of establishing whether a person has 'insight' into their state of body and mind, that is, whether they are insane. Whether they have the capacity to make specific decisions, even if they are unwise decisions.

GPs are faced with multiple requests to regulate and certify who is exempt from civil duties: exempt from appearing in court, exempt from going to school, eligible for a refund of holiday costs, eligible for a ground floor flat in social housing, able to drive, not able to drive or park in the bay closest to the entrance to the supermarket.

The medical profession is deeply woven into the fabric of social control. The medicalization of behaviour and emotions places doctors right at the heart of the regulation of passions and rational reasoning. This can be in the guise of prescribing antidepressants for anger and frustration; it can also be in the shape of forcing people into treatments under coercion and behind locked doors to ensure 'safety'. All these processes are standardized, regulated, and overseen by the law.

A woman sees a GP for back pain. At the end of the consultation, she discloses that her partner has recently become verbally abusive towards her after losing his job, and it is getting her down. She reports that their daughter has not been too affected by the situation at home and asks the GP not to record safeguarding concerns on the medical notes.

This case illustrates a commonly occurring situation in GP when loyalties are divided and decision-making is conflicted. Protecting the child and the mother is paramount, but invoking the safeguarding process – informing social services, coding concerns on the notes, etc. – often has the effect of alienating the family, who then avoid future contact with any healthcare professional once the investigation has taken place and they are no longer under surveillance. Conversely, maintaining a trusted relationship can be protective, with regular follow-up to reassess the situation. This requires the clinician to shoulder the associated risks – the risk that the situation is more dangerous than the woman has disclosed; that the child or mother will come to harm that could have been prevented; that they themselves may be subject to censure for not following the letter of the law. This is only feasible if the clinician is part of a supportive team where continuity of care is encouraged. As Victor Montori and Dominique Allwood state: 'care requires a person to notice another's human situation and to respond to it. In healthcare, that response should be safe and based on the best evidence, but also specific, and co-created with and for each patient.'[6]

Glossary of Common Terms Used in the Administration of Mental Healthcare

MHA assessment	The Mental Health Act (2005) sets out when people can be admitted to hospital without giving their consent in order to receive mental health treatment. An MHA assessment is a procedure of social administration, regulated under the MHA. It involves a registered Psychiatrist, an approved mental health professional (AMHP, a social worker with extended training), and a Section 12/2 approved GP. The assessment can be a joint procedure or carried out over a period of time in staggered episodes. The AMHP curates the procedure.
MHA Section 2	Admission to a specialized unit for further assessment where the situation is unclear. There is an appeal procedure in place to challenge decisions.
MHA Section 3	Admission to a specialized unit for treatment for up to six months, for example administration of antipsychotic drugs.
Community Treatment Order (CTO)	A CTO is an order made by a responsible clinician to give a mental health patient supervised treatment in the community after they have been in hospital. Conditions are added to the CTO which they have to follow; like having to live in a certain place, taking medication or going to appointments for treatment. It is akin to a prisoner released on licence and includes restrictions on the freedom to roam and compulsory administration of medication.

(Continued)

Glossary of Common Terms Used in the Administration of Mental Healthcare

Deprivation of Liberty Safeguard (DOLS)	If you are in a hospital or care home, your liberty can normally only be taken away if health professionals use the procedures called the Deprivation of Liberty Safeguards (DOLS). This protects you from having your liberty taken away without good reason. DOLS is linked to the assessment of mental capacity.
Mental capacity	Section 2 of the Mental Capacity Act 2005 says that 'a person lacks capacity in relation to a matter if at the material time he is unable to make a decision for himself in relation to the matter because of an impairment of, or a disturbance in the functioning of, the mind or brain'. Lacking capacity includes where your ability to make decisions is affected: <ul><li>permanently: this is where your ability to make decisions is always affected. This might be because, for example, you have a form of dementia, a learning disability, or brain injury. Or,</li><li>in the short term, this means your ability to make decisions changes from day to day. This might be because, for example, you are confused because you're on medication or because of some mental health conditions, or you are unconscious.</li></ul> Mental capacity relates to specific decisions. These can be low-level (shopping) or high-level (moving house).
Mental capacity assessment	The assessment of mental capacity assumes at baseline that the index patient has the capacity to make specific decisions. These decisions can be unwise. A professional assessment evaluates the ability to retain information and the ability to balance the pros and cons of a decision.

(*Continued*)

Glossary of Common Terms Used in the Administration of Mental Healthcare

Best interest	Sometimes health and social care professionals have to make decisions about a patient when they lack the capacity to make decisions. It involves close relatives, and for those with dementia people with lasting power of attorney. The checklist assessing the best interest includes:

- considering your wishes and feelings: both your current wishes and those you expressed before losing the capacity to make the decision, as well as any beliefs and values that are important to you;
- considering all the circumstances relevant to you, like the type of mental health problem or physical illness you have, how long it is going to last, your age, whether you would normally take this decision yourself, whether you are likely to recover capacity in the near future, and who has cared or is caring for you;
- considering whether you will have the capacity to make the decision in future and whether the decision can be put off in the short term. If you are experiencing severe mental distress, for example, will your distress ease in the near future enough to let you make your own decisions?;
- supporting your involvement in acts done for you and decisions affecting you;
- considering the views of your carers, family, or people who may have an interest in your welfare or people you have appointed to act for you.

Notes

1. Eileen Munro, *The Munro Eeview of Child Protection: Final Report, a Child-Centred System*, vol. 8062 (London: The Stationery Office, 2011).

2. Sarah Matthews, Philip O'Hare, and Jill Hemmington, *Approved Mental Health Practice: Essential Themes for Students and Practitioners* (London: Macmillan International Higher Education, 2014).

3. Lucy Series, 'Making Sense of Cheshire West', in *The Legacies of Institutionalisation: Disability, Law and Policy in the 'Deinstitutionalised' Community*, ed. C. Spivakovsky, L. Steele, and P. Weller (Oxford: Hart Publishing, 2020), https://www.ncbi.nlm.nih.gov/books/NBK559396/.

4. Emily Alison and Laurence Alison, *Rapport: The Four Ways to Read People* (New York: Random House, 2020).

5. Thomas Hobbes and Marshall Missner, *Thomas Hobbes: Leviathan (Longman Library of Primary Sources in Philosophy)* (London: Routledge, 2016).

6. Victor M. Montori and Dominique Allwood, *Careful, Kind Care Is Our Compass Out of the Pandemic Fog* (UK: British Medical Journal Publishing Group, 2022).

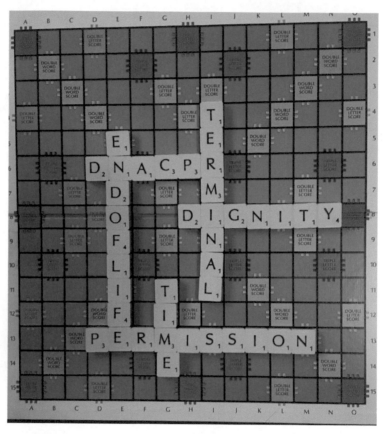

FIGURE 6.1: Scrabble 6, 'Terminal', Rupal Shah and Jens Foell, 2021.

6.
Passports for Passing: The Bureaucracy of Death

Death avoidance is not an individual failing; it's a cultural one. Facing death is not for the faint-hearted. It is far too challenging to expect that each citizen will do so on his or her own. Death acceptance is the responsibility of all death professionals – funeral directors, cemetery managers, hospital workers. It is the responsibility of those who have been tasked with creating physical and emotional environments where safe, open interaction with death and dead bodies is possible.

(Caitlin Doughty[1])

The river Styx separates Life and Death. As with any border, there must be assurance that the paperwork is correct.

(Jens, 2022)

Health services struggle and very often fail to 'create physical and emotional environments where safe, open interaction with death and dead bodies is possible'.[2] A major problem is around ceilings of care – the thorny question of when it is better to make an investment into prolonging the lives of sick people by sending them to hospital for treatment; or conversely when the time has come to acknowledge that prolonging life is no longer possible and that a different approach should be taken, whereby the investment is instead into improving quality of life by increasing care at home and possibly allowing natural death to happen. This needs a lot of discussion, organization, and administration – so ideally planning to allow death to happen and thinking about what will constitute a good death has to start early. Like home births, home deaths can be very traumatic and not every family or household is cut out to shoulder the emotional labour associated with care for the dying. Like birth plans, there are attempts to formalize plans and decisions for the end of life. But as with birth, events surrounding death are often not predictable. What constitutes a 'good' or 'natural' death is always shaped by the cultural values people attribute to death and dying. Joan Bakewell suggests 'we should talk about death', but these conversations differ widely between and within cultures.[3]

The art of living is intertwined with the art of dying. In medieval Christianity, there were textbooks giving guidance on *ars moriendi*.[4] Kathryn Mannix updated this counsel for our time in her book *With the End in Mind: How to Live and Die Well*.[5] Diagnosing dying is a process, not a one-off decision.[6] Starting a conversation about death during life is risky and prone to misinterpretation. Unfortunately, the three-letter acronym TLC (tender loving care) is often considered to be the second choice or the same as giving up – 'bravely fighting' can be a moral obligation in western culture when it comes to death[7] and obituaries talk of patients losing battles.[8] For all these reasons, talk of death comes late and good conversations are rare. They require the right relationship, the right setting, and the right timing. The structural changes we have already discussed – in particular, reduced continuity of care and reluctance to take emotional risks pose a particular challenge. Who wants to stick their head above the parapet and point out that the Emperor's New Clothes don't exist – that there are no more medical interventions which will prolong life, that trying to do so is futile and likely to cause only distress and pain to the patient and to their loved ones.

There is considerable paperwork to be completed once it has eventually been established that natural death should be allowed to happen. The river Styx separates life from death. As with any border, if you are to be allowed passage, you require the correct documentation, which must be complete and up to date. Border control at the river Styx is manned by doctors, community nurses, registrars, and funeral directors; and the DNACPR form is the passport required to cross to the other side.

In its guidance for doctors on cardiopulmonary resuscitation (CPR), the General Medical Council states:

> When someone suffers sudden cardiac or respiratory arrest, CPR attempts to restart their heart or breathing and restore their circulation. CPR interventions are invasive and include chest compressions, electric shock by an external or implanted defibrillator, injection of drugs and ventilation. If attempted promptly, CPR has a reasonable success rate in some circumstances. Generally, however, CPR has a very low success rate and the burdens and risks of CPR include harmful side effects such as rib fracture and damage to internal organs; adverse clinical outcomes such as hypoxic brain damage; and other consequences for the patient such as increased physical disability. If the use of CPR is not successful in restarting the heart or breathing, and in restoring circulation, it may mean that the patient dies in an undignified and traumatic manner.[9]

'Do Not Attempt Cardiopulmonary Resuscitation' (DNACPR) means different things to different people in different circumstances, different cultures, and different situations.

The order serves a different purpose for healthcare staff than for patients and their relatives. It may herald the beginning of the end. It can be a document allowing the healthcare professionals involved in the case to relax, because death is allowed to happen, and nobody is to be blamed if death occurs.

DNACPR can be the overt signal documenting a paradigm change: 'This patient is allowed to die.' 'This patient is sick enough to die and will not come back if the heart shuts down as part of a generalised chain reaction.' Stating this can mean that there is no hope of returning to full function anymore. It can mean that finally the suffering is almost over, and the end is near.

It is only once patients are officially on 'the pathway' leading to death and all forms about their preferred place of care and their preferred place of death have been documented by an authorized person, that death is no longer the enemy or failure. This is when the paradigm of avoidance finally shifts. Correctly filled out, the pathway includes information about people's preferences, an up-to-date 'Do Not Attempt Cardiopulmonary Resuscitation' (DNACPR) form, prescription charts, and symptom-checking charts. Then their status is changed to 'end-of-life' in handovers and clinicians are absolved from the shame and blame that otherwise would occur in the event of death. Once categorized in this way, healthcare professionals have a clear agenda, and patients are slotted into the end-of-life or palliative category in handovers and have special notes put on their electronic computer records. The obligation of the health professional to prolong life is finally waived. Instead, their role is officially to walk beside the family as a guide and a witness, along a waymarked trail. Death is allowed to happen. The presence of such an institutionally enshrined protocol of support for dying patients is the result of the efforts of the hospice movement.

Decisions about death are delicate and must be handled carefully and with caution. Patients and their families need to believe that the healthcare staff looking after them have their best interests at heart and that their motives can be held up to scrutiny. The ill-fated Liverpool Care Pathway (LCP) was introduced to the UK in the late 1990s with the intention of improving end-of-life care and was further refined over the next 15 years until it was abruptly withdrawn in 2014 under a cloud of negative publicity and mistrust. Despite all its virtuous aspirations, implementation of the LCP in hospitals led to negative outcomes. 'Relatives and carers felt that they had been "railroaded" into agreeing to put the patient on a one-way escalator', wrote the editors of the Independent Review of the LCP.[10] The stories in this book explore the dynamics between virtuous bureaucratic aspirations, their embodiment in organizational protocols and institutionalized ways of operating. The discretionary space of frontline workers, street-level bureaucrats, can be occupied by the letter or the spirit of the regulatory framework.

The stories are told from the perspective of general practice (within normal working hours and Out-of-Hours). A role of the GP described in John Berger's *A Fortunate Man* is that of 'Familiar of death' – the professional familiar of death and dying, embedded in the community, not only familiar with both patients' lives and families, but also with the biological process of dying and its medico-political administration.[11] Being familiar involves pastoral care, genuine doctoring, handling living and dead bodies, and the social administration of death and dying.

Of utmost relevance to those of us working in primary care is that although death marks the end of the story for the patient, it is simply a chapter in the life book of those they leave behind – who are often registered at the same practice. What follows for the family is heavily coloured by the memory of how the loved one died.

The stories in this chapter are located in the twilight zone, which intersects the paradigms of defying or accepting death.

A Family Man

I remember their large, airy flat with its river views. I had been there before, but to see her, not him.

I knew Eve well, she saw me for her osteoporosis and for her painful feet which were the legacy of a different chapter of her life. I advised her periodically to stop wearing high heels and she ignored me. She had danced professionally as a younger woman and you could still catch a trace of those old rhythms when she walked. She chose Henry over her dancing, the two great loves of her life. Henry was better known to a colleague of mine at the practice. In the past year or two, his health had been steadily declining. This downward trajectory had started a couple of years back when he suffered from a stroke which had left him with some residual weakness. He had since developed troublesome leg ulcers which needed regular dressings by our practice nurses. His mobility was also limited by his heart, which wasn't pumping as well as it should have been. Once a keen walker, he had had no choice but to start using a wheelchair. It was tricky for Eve to manoeuvre this wheelchair into the lift when they wanted to go out, but she had been just about managing. She had declined carers, preferring to look after Henry herself.

Sometimes, it is hard to step back and take an overview of a patient like Henry, who has been deteriorating slowly; and to realize how bad their prognosis is – worse than it is for some types of cancer. Henry was dying, though slowly. Eve knew it, Henry too, and so did I, though none of us was able to name what was happening and face it head-on. Nothing new had happened; there were no terrible new diagnoses; this was simply an old man whose life force was gradually trickling away. It is difficult to predict how long someone in Henry's situation may have left to live – but the question that palliative care services suggest we ask ourselves is, 'Would I be surprised if this patient were to die within the next year?', when considering end-of-life conversations.

The point of these difficult conversations is to ask questions about how someone would like to be cared for as they approach death, what they want and what they don't want. For example, whether they would like to be resuscitated with chest compressions and defibrillation should they have a cardiac arrest (this is very unlikely to be successful for someone like Henry and in the main, only causes unnecessary distress); where they would like to spend their final days, at home, in a hospital, or in a hospice; what the threshold of treatment should be if they were to deteriorate; and whether they want to write a legally binding advance decision to refuse treatment (ADRT).

It isn't really that easy though when someone is dying but doesn't have a disease label which medically legitimizes their prognosis. Cancer is linked in our collective psyche with death; and doctors and nurses are implicitly given permission to accept that this is the eventual destination when conventional treatments fail, so the task is to make the journey easier, not to alter the end destination.

When someone doesn't have cancer but instead has a chronic disease or several chronic diseases, it is less clear-cut. In cases like Henry's, where the decline is gradual and subtle, doctors and nurses can be reluctant to talk about what is happening and to notice the bigger picture, we become ostriches, burying our heads in the sand. There are often a series of events in the last years of life, which may be a reflection of this decline rather than being causative – chest infections, urine infections, and falls are the markers which signpost the path that someone like Henry is on. And each infection, every fall is treated. But it is rare for someone clinical to ask, 'What does this mean for you and for your family?'; 'How can I help you to preserve your dignity and autonomy?'; 'What do you want from the health service and what don't you want?'

We are afraid of the fallout and we doubt ourselves. These are difficult questions to ask and might not be welcome. Are they permitted, are we allowed to ask them? What is our role here – is it even our business? Are we bureaucrats or advocates?

Before we realize, it is too late to ask someone what they want because they no longer have the ability to tell us.

Although we didn't have a DNACPR form in place, Eve was legally recognized as Henry's attorney, meaning that should he lose capacity, she had the ability to make decisions on his behalf. A power-of-attorney is a legal authorization made by the donor (in this case Henry) to their attorney to give them the power to make decisions for them in the event of loss of capacity. This authorization can be for financial affairs and/or health matters. Having a power-of-attorney in place gave Eve the legal ability to make decisions about Henry's health when he could no longer make them himself. Its existence turned out to be important in influencing the subsequent turn of events.

Henry's slow deterioration came to a head one cold, grey Friday evening at the start of March, with winter still lingering in the air. Eve phoned the surgery, distraught that he was struggling to breathe. She refused to call an ambulance, so I visited after my evening surgery.

I knew as soon as I entered their bedroom that the situation was bad. Henry was ashen, propped up in bed, gasping for breath. He was conscious, but couldn't manage more than a few words. Examining him, it was clear that his heart condition had worsened and that he was in acute heart failure, with fluid building up in his lungs and preventing him from breathing. I told Eve that he needed admission to hospital and that I would arrange an ambulance. Eve looked at me and simply shook her head. She walked over to Henry and held his hand. 'We don't want that, thank you, Roo', she said. 'Please can you just make him comfortable?'

All Henry could add in short, painful gasps was 'Eve knows what to do for the best'. He held onto his wife's hand as if he was her child instead of her husband.

I explained to Eve that Henry might not survive if he stayed at home, and that the medicines I could prescribe to help relieve his symptoms might not be enough to save him. Eve told me that she understood, but wouldn't change her mind. She didn't want her final memories of Henry after all the decades of being together to be of him in a hospital ward, surrounded by strangers and the accoutrements of medicine instead of the mementoes of the life they had lived together. She wanted to remember him at home where he belonged. Their two adult daughters and son were already making their way over to the flat along with the grandchildren – and Eve intended that they should spend the rest of the evening together, taking it in turns to be with Henry. She wanted me to make sure he was comfortable and well enough to be able to say his goodbyes peacefully. I prescribed a diuretic to help offload the extra fluid building up in his lungs and a low dose of morphine to help with his breathing and pain. The memory of this Friday home visit still affects me because I was making decisions I don't normally make alone.

1. I decided that Henry didn't have the capacity to understand what his options were.
2. I thought that Eve should be the one to decide on his behalf.
3. I decided that prolonging Henry's life was probably not the most important consideration here.

I knew there was no DNACPR form and that this was not clear-cut. Echoes of Harold Shipman rung in my ears – it felt like a knife edge and I was frightened of being accused of being negligent or of expediting Henry's death.

In the end, Henry lasted another week before dying at home with Eve by his side, having said goodbye to each of his children.

It is hard to think about dying in the midst of life, but perhaps it's something we should be thinking about more than is the case now. My friend and colleague at the surgery who was Palliative Care Lead for many years put it this way: 'we need to talk more about death, because it has almost disappeared from our daily life'. It has been brought into the realm and governance of medicine.

Eve was a remarkable woman, who was able to understand the harm that would have resulted from Henry being admitted to hospital and of being denied those last days with him. In my experience, the way in which someone dies can have a significant effect on how their loved ones cope with their loss. Even though Eve grieved when Henry died, she was able to recover and had the feeling that his wishes had been respected until the very end, that she had done her duty and not allowed herself to be swayed from what she knew was right. In the end, Henry's death was in keeping with his life. He always was a family man.

Psychogeographies of Grief
70s TV Classics and Tender Loving Care

Crows Gold is the title of a Swedish TV programme I (Jens)
watched as a child. It is a suspense story featuring children finding
gold in a Swedish quarry town. I found it eerie, truly nail-biting.
And I remember the vibe of the film and the town, with the quarry
towering over the scene.

I am getting similar vibes from Penmaenmawr. The mountain
dividing Llanfairfechan and Penmaenmawr, the two towns our
practice serves, looks like the moon. Its surface is dark and rugged,
with terraces and conveyor belts and re-conservation and landslide
protection devices.

There is a huge clock mounted on the mountain. Yes, on the
mountain, not on a church tower. It used to serve the purpose of
summoning the quarry workers to duty.

The West of Penmaenmawr is dominated by the economy and
ecology of the quarry. The terraces found here were the prototypes
for the iconic British working-class terraced house – and we do our
home visits in this area. Penmaenmawr-stones were used in the
British railway industry. Industrialization, fuelled by the railways,
relied on the stones provided by this mountain, excavated by its
workers. The industrial history of the quarry has left its imprint on
Penmaenmawr.

Over the years, an invisible network of psychoactive spots
of drama and grief has built up in my memory. These are the
locations where lives ended, care commitments transformed into
either an eternally open wound or a sublime act of passion, where
lives have stopped, and lives have gone on.

There was a call-back. The wife of Dave was the caller, and
she was very, very angry. I could see that secondary care had had
problems in negotiating a palliative strategy with Dave and his
wife. So, the gastroenterologists asked the GP to break bad news/
undertake difficult negotiations, whatever we choose to call such
conversations.

And it must have gone wrong. The Senior Partner, known for
her compassion, volunteered for the job, and I could see how it
had not worked. I could see wife G being angry, she employed
military metaphors, 'He is a fighter'. So, talking about what to
do in the case of him dying/his heart ceasing to beat (whether
or not to resuscitate) did not start on a shared interpretation of

his state. In this home visit, I was not pushy (for 'closure', the administration of dying, DNACPR, etc.) but I said I would refer to palliative care to get help with symptom relief. It did not work. She put the phone down on the palliative care nurse. I had thought it would help – he was not drinking enough, he was not eating, he had problems evacuating his bowels, and everything abdominal was an issue.

I could see that this case was going to be stuck. The district nurse had been sent home. Everything was wrong. Anger, frustration. I don't like the word 'denial' – who am I to say that somebody accepts or does not accept what is seen as the 'truth'.[12] However, it was clear that the end was not far away.

He had a crisis, a chest infection, and got admitted to hospital. I contacted the ward; I contacted the hospital palliative care team. I could see from the notes that the medical team struggled with the wife. Eventually, Dave got discharged. As expected, the transfer to 'the community' aka home, included communication mishaps. Palliative care had not been involved. The DNACPR form had not been sent over. District nurses did not want to visit the house without having reassurance that they would not have to deliver CPR in case he died, which was very likely to happen. This conflict led me, the GP, to step into this linguistically volatile territory. We agreed on regular visits and I got used to walking up the sideway to the cottage, to the quarry environment, almost like Tarkowski's *Stalker*. The district nurses and I kept in contact with brief communications and, whilst on duty elsewhere on the weekend, I got the message that he had passed away in the early hours one Sunday morning.

As I had promised his wife on Saturday that I would be back on Monday, I returned to their home. I knew the much-feared moment had happened over the weekend. How was she getting on? In our model, death does not bring closure. Death is the opening to yet another episode – with loved ones, with loving ones. The focus is always on the dying but also on the carers. They are the next to be seen. We then deal better with everybody, with his wife, his daughter, and his friends. Palliative care in primary care is not about the index individual. We invest in the next death when this one is over. This is the difference between primary and secondary care. The never-ending story. The perpetual, daily grind. When I visited his wife the day after Dave's body left the cottage, she said,

'Sorry I have been a bitch'. Crocuses were blossoming in the shade of the trees. Life goes on.

Down the road is 'Ponderosa'. Houses in North Wales can have imaginative names. This house makes me think of the *Waltons and of Bonanza*, another 1970s TV series. The daughter called me to attend to her mother. The scenario was a geriatric classic.

Mrs. M spends most time of the day on her chair. At times she sleeps on the chair. She has four pillows in her bed and gets breathless at night. This breathlessness makes her panicky. The daughter thinks about buying her a nebulizer machine for her lungs but the story strongly suggests heart failure. With these concepts in mind, I set out for Ponderosa.

The visit consisted of two encounters. One was the centre-stage encounter. Mrs. M sits in the chair, and I am on the floor and examine the legs, prod their consistency and texture, listen to her chest, feel her abdomen, put a pulse oximeter on her finger, and take blood from her elbow crease. And I think ahead: 'Start water tablets', 'organise follow up', 'heart failure clinic', and further down the line, deteriorating heart failure, palliative care, death.

She blankly refuses to go to the hospital, where all investigations could be done in one go. The state of the house tells me that she is not able to maintain it any more. Her life has condensed to the chair. The daughter hovers around me and I sense how anxious she is about her mother. She tells me that her mother avoided calling the GP for quite some time. Now, something has to happen. And it happens.

'Think big', 'Think ahead', I think, 'DNACPR', I am slightly pushy in setting the scene for what will come at some point in the future. I say that in my other role as a GP in the Out-of-Hours service, I often enter such scenes at crisis point, and then dramatic decisions have to be made when patients no longer have the capacity to do so. In my patch, I want to avoid this. I do not fill in any forms or take notes, but invite Mrs. M and her daughter to talk about death.

So far so good, something will happen now, I have set things in motion. I prescribe diuretics and will make the necessary referrals once back at the practice.

On the way out I ask the daughter how she is. This invitation for the daughter to speak independently outside her mother's presence brings out tears. Six years ago, the husband/father died, 'she never got over it and maybe never will'. I learn that the husband had cancer and was nursed at home. It was the end of an episode in one way, but I am now dealing with the sequelae in another life.

I am heading back to the practice and pass by the place where the man I called Charles Bronson was nursed by his wife with never-ending, tender loving care. He had the privilege or luxury of dying at home, in his own environment, with his music in the background and a poster of Charles Bronson on the wall.

I saw his wife recently. Half a year later, she made an appointment with me to review all the sinister symptoms she was sensing in her own body. Facing death in a loved one changes the body we inhabit into an eerie environment. And yet again the interpretive skills of the GP as a mediator between the lived body and higher powers are bitterly needed. This is not pastoral care, it is a combination of a biomedical check-up, soul searching, and coaching.

Death in the Time of a Pandemic
Being able to make decisions in advance about death depends on there being realistic options to choose from and on people having the capacity to make the choices they are being asked to make. The question of how and when we make these decisions was thrown into sharp relief by the COVID-19 pandemic.

At the height of the crisis, hospitals near our practice in London had the air of battle zones. Intensive care facilities had been expanded as much as possible, for example by converting operating theatres and daycare facilities into makeshift Intensive Treatment Units (ITUs). Emergency departments were filled with patients struggling to breathe. All elective work was on hold or was being done virtually. And the brutal reality was that before the vaccination programme was rolled out, patients with COVID-19 who became ill enough to need ITU admission had a very poor prognosis even if they were mechanically ventilated. The chances of survival were even lower for older people and those with chronic diseases.

Hospital wasn't necessarily a good place to be. It meant being separated from family, who might not be allowed to visit – hospitals were keeping visitors to a bare minimum. Adult in-patients were only allowed a visitor if they took a turn for the worse. Dying alone in a hospital seemed to be a worse alternative for some than staying at home, even if this did expedite death. Whether to admit people over the age of 65 to critical care units was, for a brief period, partly determined by the use of a clinical frailty score, whereby critical care admission was not guaranteed for patients who were considered to be mildly frail or worse (meaning that they routinely needed help with more complicated daily living activities such as managing finances and heavy housework). These factors have always implicitly played into decision-making processes, but to make explicit the need to consider population as well as individual benefit was new.

In other words, the COVID-19 pandemic meant a shift away from doing the best for the individual patient being treated to considering what would bring the greatest benefit to the greatest number – although arguably, this is unknowable and at best is an educated guess.

As GPs, we were asked to have discussions with our frailer patients about what they would like to do if they fell ill with the virus and had the choice of whether or not to go to hospital. An associated question was about resuscitation decisions, that is whether people wanted to be actively resuscitated. CPR has a very low success rate overall, particularly in people who are elderly with underlying chronic illnesses. Resuscitation guidelines changed with the advent of coronavirus, with mouth-to-mouth resuscitation no longer recommended and where possible, it was advised that defibrillation should be attempted before chest compressions. Some areas stopped performing manual CPR altogether because of the high risk of viral spread and the low chance of success. Resuscitating someone usually entails an ITU admission afterwards, if it works – at the height of the pandemic, this was of course especially difficult.

There is much to be said about the logic of what was asked of GPs. Intensive interventions were unlikely to work and might result in more harm than good, including the possibility of a lonely, frightening death in hospital. But there was a stark undertone related to rationing, something which we are not used to addressing so explicitly. The negative publicity which followed is proof that these conversations have to be handled with care. Newspaper headlines told stories of patients being sent letters by their GPs asking them to make decisions about whether they wanted to be resuscitated. Although there were clear benefits of considering carefully which option was the best of a bad bunch, we were being asked to contact our frailest patients not only for their benefit, but also for the benefit of everyone else so that limited resources wouldn't be 'wasted'. This is a brutal message to hear from your family doctor. It was further complicated by other factors. Firstly, these frail, vulnerable patients were being asked to self-isolate, which usually meant limited contact with their family and friends. Not everyone had the ability or technology to access the virtual ways of keeping in touch which have become so well established now.

The psychological effect of this isolation and change in routine for people who were already scared was devastating. It meant that someone who was managing reasonably well with daily or weekly visits from a son or daughter and a friendly neighbour who popped in a couple of times a week to do shopping now had almost no social contact. Even carers were limiting contact to the very essentials of what needed to be done and should have been wearing a mask, apron and goggles when they did come. Often poor hearing made telephone conversations difficult, further heightening isolation. The result was that people whom I would previously have judged as having no significant mental impairment became disorientated and distressed.

We were having to contact people who were in this state of mind not in person but by telephone. It would have been easier to make the decision not to admit to hospital if there had been adequate end-of-life care in the community. In our locality, even without coronavirus there had long been a shortage of community nursing staff. During the pandemic, many staff members were off work either due to illness (people with any respiratory symptoms, even if only mild were asked to stay away from work) or because they had to self-isolate due to underlying health conditions or contact with a symptomatic family member. The local hospice was full, similarly understaffed and struggling to accept any new referrals. So offering the option of high-quality end-of-life care at home or in the community seemed to be a promise that we couldn't fulfil.

'Many of us oldies accept we are going to die and for some of us COVID-19 will be a short cut. What we're really scared about is dying without connection and saying proper

goodbyes.' This was a tweet from Richard Lehman, retired GP and academic.

These emotive words summarize the conundrum with which we were faced. Good end-of-life care is all about connection – with family, friends, clinicians, and carers looking after you. A chance to say goodbye and to look back on the life you have lived surrounded by the people who have meant the most to you. The need to limit the spread of the virus made this connection almost impossible, as families and friends were forced to stay away from one another, and clinicians started working by telephone or video call where feasible.

I remember one particular consultation vividly because it was so heartbreaking. I telephoned an elderly man whose wife I knew well, because we had received notification that she had been admitted to hospital. It turned out that the admission had been a couple of weeks ago and was because she had developed a urine infection. This happened at the end of February 2020, just before the number of cases of virus started to rise exponentially. Tragically, she contracted COVID-19 whilst in hospital and because of this, she was still an in-patient at the time I rang. Her husband sobbed on the phone to me, distraught that he wasn't able to see her, comfort her, or hold her hand. She was too confused to speak to him on the phone and he didn't understand what was happening to her, whether she would live or die. He was in a state of utter panic, not going out anywhere (as the government had advised) and living on food which his kind neighbours and community volunteers delivered to him. He didn't have an internet connection and was utterly isolated and bewildered. 'We've been married for 55 years. I don't remember life without her. I just want her back. I'm only not slitting my wrists in case she comes home.'

Sometimes, people chose to put themselves at risk to protect older, beloved family members. We had one couple in their mid 90s registered at the practice, Harold and Rona Collins. Mrs. Collins was frail, with moderately severe Alzheimer's, but no other physical ailments. Her husband was relatively well considering his age, other than suffering from chronic obstructive pulmonary disease, a result of four decades of smoking in his younger days. He had recently been started on home oxygen to help with the breathlessness he suffered as a result of his illness. He had stayed active and engaged with life until almost the end, and it had been a huge blow to him when his shortness of breath meant he could no longer go for his daily walk. Sadly, he was the first of the pair to fall ill. He was admitted to hospital where he died the next day, of COVID-19-related pneumonia. When his wife developed a fever two days later, their older daughter, herself in her 70s left her home in Kent and moved in with her mother against all official advice. Although the couple had carers who came in twice a day, it was the daughter who sat with her mother, holding her, encouraging her to take sips of water and soup, and cleaning the soiled sheets and underwear. With the help of her deceased husband's home oxygen, pain-killing medication, and her daughter's devotion, Rona was able to stay at home, where she too passed away a week later.

Although her daughter used a mask and gloves as much as she could, she almost certainly would have caught the virus herself. I hope that she fared better from it than her mother and father and that if she did become ill, she had someone to look after her. She told me that she had to do what she did because she couldn't have carried on living, knowing that her mother had died alone.

These decisions are extraordinary ones to have to make. Despite the 750,000 strong army of National Health Service volunteers recruited during the crisis, in the end, families had to make choices which usually we are shielded from in western society. When contact between strangers is not possible, caregiving falls to the ones who love you.

Do Not Attempt Resurrection

Once I received a complaint stating that I mentioned the word 'death' three times in consultation with a patient and their family about terminal care. This is another take on the D word.

The Saturday Out-of-Hours shift started with an ambulance call: the crew had been called to a 90-year-old woman who refused to go to hospital. She was weak and frail, but otherwise active and alert.

She was dehydrated from vomiting. Until two days ago she had been fully independent.

In the driveway of her sheltered bungalow, I could see her small car.

'Are you like Prince Philip?', I teased her.

'How dare you!', she replied. 'I wear my seatbelt and I always drive very carefully.'

I could see, don't mess with her. She knows what she wants. And she wanted to stay at home, in her home, her castle. But she was clearly not well, she had bouts of vomiting. The vomit was brownish. It did not smell of faeces, but it was brown.

In medical school students have to learn to distinguish between the different types of vomiting: when it is 'coffee ground' indicating a haemorrhage of blood from the stomach and when it is 'faecal', indicating a bowel obstruction. Arcane, archaic knowledge.

This time, it was not the archetypal or textbook appearance of vomit that you get with internal bleeding, it was an in-between version.

I followed her wishes and said, 'Ok, I can give you anti-sickness medication and arrange for more input, but basically, you should go to hospital'.

'No.'

She said, 'No!'

I said, 'I respect your determination and wishes, and I will come back tomorrow to check how you are'.

The next day, she still looked the same. Dry, weak. There was a slight smell of urine. I noted the Holy Bible next to her bed. I liked her resolve and softened my manner. This time we could communicate better. After prolonged negotiations with the hospital ('She has to go to A&E ... we have no beds on the medical admission ward ... she would end up being more or less unsupervised on the corridor.') I was able to arrange a place in Eryri, the local cottage hospital.

A halfway house.

I said I would follow her there and formally arrange for her admission.

When I saw her in her new, hospitalized situation she was more stable, but still retching brownish vomit. Her abdomen was distended. Her veins were so brittle and empty that I could not insert an intravenous cannula. The nurses were not happy about having her there, and she was too unwell for them to manage her. I decided that she needed to be admitted under the surgical team in the local district general hospital. When we discussed this, she said to me, 'I do not want to be resurrected'.

In my mind I smiled, no return from the dead.

I knew that she did not want to go to hospital; she feared that it would be a one-way ticket, no return. And she might be right. Even if there was an operable cause for her bowel obstruction, I had my doubts about whether she would be fit enough to survive the surgery.

The case kept on occupying my mind. Yes, I went along with her directions; I respected her capacity, which may have lost valuable time. But maybe she knew what she was doing and wanted to avoid the inevitable. I assisted her for a day in ostrich mode.

I also noted what a difference it made to see her when I was a guest in her home compared to seeing her wearing a gown and surrounded by all the medical paraphernalia in a hospital environment, where the balance of power no longer tipped in her favour.

I checked out what happened ....

I phoned the surgical ward: she was alive ... good news; had been admitted, good news; and they didn't want to tell me more for confidentiality reasons ....

So, I went up to see her. It was nice to see her again. We talked briefly. She was weak.

I learnt later that the scan showed that the cause of the bowel obstruction was a strangulated hernia.

The surgical team decided to operate on her.

She died the day after the operation.

To Have and to Hold – Journey's End

I had witnessed Lily's gradual deterioration over several years.

By the end, she couldn't make it to the surgery any longer, so when we saw each other, it was in her home.

When she couldn't stand because of the arthritis or breathe because of her failing heart or see because of her macular degeneration, her husband Ed carried her from the bedroom they shared, relocated to the ground floor, to the breakfast table every morning and back again at night. She weighed as much as him, but he managed. He fed her, cooked for her, changed her pads, and creamed her legs several times a day, which were swollen with lymphoedema. Their house was always filled with family members every time I went there. Lily was proud of her children, grandchildren, and great-grandchildren. The fridge was kept well stocked with chocolate biscuits in case any of them popped over.

Her death from pneumonia was unexpected; yet in another way, it was amazing that she lived as long as she did. She had been feeling unwell for a couple of days with a cold and cough and went to bed on Friday evening earlier than usual. She was unrousable in the morning.

It took a long time for Ed to come to terms with her death. He had been the one who had kept her alive for years more than I would ever have predicted. His care and attention to detail were infinitely more effective than anything I could hope to do.

He still misses the small things. When she was alive, he used to make a flask of tea each morning for her to sip on over the next few hours while she did her crosswords. When she died, it was the hardest thing for him to remember to stop doing this. In the end, the only way was to throw away the flask.

Lily had a complicated medical history with virtually no part of her body remaining unaffected by illness by the end. Other patients in her situation end up being under the care of several specialist clinics. These appointments can occur with such frequency that they take on a life of their own and become almost the means as well as the end. Each clinic visit leads to further investigations, follow-up after changes in medications, suggestions of interventions which then cause side effects and more appointments. I am not sure whether being under different specialist teams would have prolonged Lily's life or not, but my opinion is that it wouldn't have. The real success in her case was that she was able to live her life on her terms. I could help sometimes to make her symptoms more bearable, but my role was always a drop in the ocean compared to the role of her family, her friends, and her own spirit. Even when things were really difficult, Ed made it clear that he didn't want extra help or respite, and that his place was by Lily's side.

When I look back, I think that perhaps one of the more important things I did was to prevent too many referrals and too much intervention. It didn't always feel comfortable – it was unusual for Lily not to be seeing various specialists given her medical situation. The rise of litigation has led to doctors practising defensively so that when I make a decision to refer or investigate, my worry about being complained against feeds into this decision-making. What I choose is therefore not always with my patient's best interests in mind. It is a subject we don't talk about as often as we should.

It is clear that it was Ed's devotion to her that kept Lily alive for so many more years than we might have expected.

A healthcare assistant who had been on leave when Lily eventually passed away burst into tears when she found out the news a few months later. I don't know why they had this effect on all of us. Perhaps they represented an ideal of what marriage can be, what we all aspire to. Not only because I want to be looked after as Lily was, but perhaps I also want to be like Ed, who was so happy to care for her because he loved her.

Dying from Disgust
Food and Drink Refusal in End-Stage Dementia

Handover, Sunday morning in Out-of-Hours. I have just started my shift and the night doctor apologizes for having arranged a home visit for me. Unfortunately, this visit is far, far away; it takes an hour to get to the dementia care home, where a carer asked for help in the middle of the night.

Carers are concerned about Mrs. H. She refuses fluids. She pushes the feeding hands away, turns her head away, and spits the fluid out. This is unusual. This is new. Something needs to happen. Can't go on like this.

My colleague tried to arrange hospital admission (dehydration!), but the ambulance system was overwhelmed, and she was told that everything that is NOT immediately life-threatening will have to wait, six hours or even more.

What is 'immediately life threatening'?

I start to prepare for the visit and call the regional maxillofacial department. Yes, they would be able to see her, if there is an acute dental abscess that needs surgical input. There are options. And the consequences of oral pain and an abscess can indeed be life-threatening: sepsis and dehydration can occur.

This is a frail and vulnerable person.

When I arrive at the care home, two carers are in attendance. The patient is in bed. 'She does not like men', they warn me. She is thin. Next to the bed is a collection of closed water bottles and a beaker containing tea. She is wearing an incontinence pad. She looks scared. I can see that there is a trusted bond between her and the carers. They can read her and even though she can't communicate her needs verbally, they know her behavioural cues.

My task is to assess the situation. I must examine the mouth and find a reason to explain the fact that she refuses all drinks. Does she refuse because of a particular taste? Is she experiencing disgust? But what is it that makes plain water disgusting? Or is this part of a different and bigger story?

The fact is that the status quo is not an option.

It is difficult to examine her mouth. It needs a lot of coaxing, like with a child. I don't see or feel a dental abscess, there is no pus, and the tonsils and throat look like other throats in this age group. She is not feverish. There are no swollen lymph nodes. The teeth and gums look like they need a deep clean. How can this be done in somebody with dementia who does not let people near her?

The carers say they give her mouth care on a daily basis. They do what they can.

Then the patient throws herself on the bed and cries, 'I want to die'.

What is going on here?

If she stays here and does not drink any water, she WILL die.

If she goes to hospital, the nurses there will not be able to read her, so admitting her could be construed as an act of relational violence. Meanwhile, I don't see a simple reason that would explain her refusal to drink ANY fluid.

Is it the infection of her gums that changes her sense of taste? And if this is the case, what can be done about it? Or is it the progression of her dementia that affects so many bodily functions?

I must convene an ad hoc best-interest meeting.

We go to the office, and I call the daughter. The daughter says that this taste thing has been going on for a while, ever since Christmas. It started with food, now it's moved on to fluids, even her favourite, tea with milk and sugar gets rejected.

And that she is fed up, 'She is giving up'. What about a dentist? 'There is a dentist, but last time they were quite harsh and dismissive to her.'

There is a DNACPR order in her files. But is this a matter of death?

Maybe yes.

What if?

I need to call a friend. I am stuck and in need of advice.

I tell the daughter that I will call a dentist friend who has experience in dealing with vulnerable people with learning disabilities. When I do, my friend's advice is that other causes need to be explored and that mouth care is important, even if done with a simple moist cotton gauze.

The carers tell me how much they like the patient, 'like a family member'. They are distressed to see her going downhill and want to do everything to improve the situation.

I call the daughter again.

We establish the facts and the choices regarding a decision.

She does NOT have the capacity to make decisions about a) going to the hospital and b) refusing fluids.

However, she has said several times that she does not want to go to hospital and very likely, hospital would not be a better place for her.

She has also become very frail, skin and bones, and her dementia has got worse during lockdown.

We are on the cusp of a difficult situation. A different interpretation of this seemingly easy dilemma (fluid refusal) has turned into a moment of a possible paradigm change.

If this is crunch time and she is about to die, should she be allowed to die?

If so, and she is dying and is allowed to die, the carers who like or even love her could carry on caring with the knowledge that they have done everything in their power for her.

We arrange that the daughter will come the next day and will make an appointment with the local dentist. The carers will carry on caring and carry out as much mouth care as they can.

Possible negligence (is this reversible?) vs. best personal care sit next to each other on the cusp of this decision.

And I have been invited to decide about the wisest thing to do.

One choice is to decide that the status quo is indeed an option.

When I return to the car, the driver remonstrates that this visit took one hour and twenty minutes. 'What were you DOING, doctor!?'

Yes, what was I doing?

I called the home two days later. The dentist confirmed the status quo has continued and that he has added a spray to the mouth care. It looks as though her life is coming to an end and all people involved in her care are keeping her as comfortable as possible. And death is going to be allowed to happen.

I was left wondering what exactly is happening. Is it disease progression or the process of dying itself (refusing food, refusing a drink, curling up), or has the foul mouth changed her sense of taste and it is disgust that will eventually kill her?

Three weeks later, I called again. I recognized the carer's voice who answered the phone. He told me that she passed away last week and that they, the carers, have been invited to attend the funeral. He said the family were heavily involved in her terminal care. They made it clear, that in case she gets worse, she should NOT go to hospital. This is what she wanted after her husband died in hospital.

Her wishes came true. She was allowed to end her life where and how she wanted her life to end.

In retrospect, I think that I attended during a watershed moment – the paradigm change from '*Crisis*'. needs hospital admission, something needs to be done and if this does not happen, the caring staff and family will be held accountable and will feel guilty and feel the need to protect their engagement and reputation' to 'is allowed to die and it is ok, our duty of care includes care for the dying'.

When thinking about the differences between primary care and secondary care, I realize that when GPs refer terminally ill patients to hospital, they often do so in order to get somebody else (a 'higher authority') to tell the patient that the options for curative approaches are running out. And the hospital clinicians focus on self-management and acceptance. Maybe it has to be this way because the statement 'this door is closed' has to come from people high up in the symbolic order of medical hierarchies. However, this approach is not logical and is counterintuitive given that it is the primary care clinicians who know the patient and their family best – in the realm of death, the boundaries of what medicine can and can*not* do are configured in the wrong way. Helping the ones you cannot help (in the core medical, curative paradigm) is outsourced to hospices or home-based care. And the decision NOT to go to secondary care implies acceptance of death.

Of course, these decisions may change and get revoked, as in any relationship, the yes and no change over time.

I also realize again that the maps which structure our decision-making space are derived from secondary care data. Which means that they often do not make sense in a primary care environment.

'Actively Dying' – The Politics of Access

'Actively dying' (and whether or not someone is classified as such) is yet another category that separates levels of service provision, privileges, and entitlements patients can expect.

Recently, I was looking after two people with motor neurone disease. One had a slowly progressing variant and was approaching the very end of his disease trajectory, also the end of his life. His advanced statement of wishes confirmed that his preferred place of care was home, but his preferred place of death was the hospice. He used to fundraise for the hospice and was well-known in the village. A character. My colleagues remember him sitting in his wheelchair outside the pub.

When the end appeared to be imminent, he spent a considerable time in the hospice but did not die after all. Therefore, the hospice sent him to a residential home, but clearly, he was too ill to cope there – he was bedbound and had to be fed through a tube directly into his stomach, bypassing his gullet where his inability to swallow would have caused a risk of aspiration. He needed around-the-clock care. Carers struggled, he had a syringe driver going and the doses of medications required were escalating.

I tried desperately to get him back into the hospice, but the people in charge of bed allocation said, 'there are no beds'. I knew this was not true because one of our patients had recently died there. There was no bed for *him*. The administrator justified her decision by telling me that beds are only available for people who are 'actively dying', which he is not. I asked how she could tell. She didn't answer but instead told me that there was a place in a nursing home which would be perfect. Unfortunately, he declined this offer. Stalemate. A summit was convened, and a representative of the palliative team and the district nursing team convinced the patient that the nursing home would be able to provide better care than he was getting currently. He accepted. I helped with the logistics and made sure the paperwork was up-to-date and there were enough drugs for his syringe driver.

The next day the district nurse told me, 'he died two hours after having arrived in the nursing home, he was gasping for breath on the way'.

The manager of the residential home wrote an angry letter to the hospice, outlining the promises which had been broken. The justification for not allowing him back was that he didn't fit the category 'actively dying'.

This difficult categorization recently affected another patient with the same condition. Mrs. T is fearfully awaiting her imminent death. Fearfully, because she fears her mode of dying. She has a fulminant, progressive version of motor neurone disease. As usual, things come to a head on Friday, with the deadline for 9–5 services approaching. She is unwell, cannot settle, has abdominal pain and increasing problems swallowing. All of a sudden, the question about hydration, usually discussed in advance with specialist services, becomes *my* question.

Should she go to hospital, where she could have a nasogastric tube inserted, a tube from her nose to her stomach so she can receive fluid to stop her dying from dehydration? But being admitted to hospital means no visits from relatives in these COVID-19 days.

The hospital doctor confirms that Mrs. T will not be able to have visitors if admitted. The only exception would be if she were 'actively dying'. Getting a nasogastric tube inserted does not constitute active dying. I hear in the tremble of the doctor's voice how uncomfortable she is in defending this boundary.

My voice becomes cold, and I say I understand her line of command, the protocols, etc., and that I will discuss the case with the family. The husband is upset. Events are heading towards an awful climax. They are expecting their children to come over soon, probably for the last time. And the question of hydration remains unsolved. Ideally, it would happen in her own home, but district nurses do not place subcutaneous drips in the community.

I call the palliative care consultant and luckily, I am able to have a productive, professional conversation with her. We confirm that the hospital is not the preferred option, and we should try to deliver services to her home. She says that district nurses can administer subcutaneous infusions under hospital instructions if the relatives can pick up the infusion bags from the hospital. There are plenty of phone calls backwards and forwards. It takes such a long time that the husband offers to give me and my bicycle a lift in the car he has bought to transport his wife in

> Plan - for end of life in IPU. Ongoing support for family.
> Performance score - dying. Phase of illness (AKPS) 10%

FIGURE 6.2: The categorization of death and dying – detail from a clinic letter from palliative care. Jens Foell, 2022.

her wheelchair, 'the most useless purchase I ever made' because she only managed maybe one or two trips before becoming bedbound.

What does the 'active' in 'actively' dying mean, and what is the difference between this and passively dying? Can the criteria be refined, and the boundaries of the classification be more clearly defined?

Going back to the theme of street-level bureaucracy, there are boundary categories everywhere, and the more closely you work with these categories, the more aware you become of their arbitrariness. What is immediate in the threat to life, what makes dying active?

A Crushing End
Border Control in Higher Pastures
A local nursing home is called Higher Pastures. I am informed that a patient died very soon after arriving there. He must have experienced a cardiac event. Staff reacted and called 999, paramedics did what they were supposed to do and worked hard on him. His chest was compressed, his ribs were broken, his heart was shocked, and he even regained a pulse for a while, but eventually, this was futile and death was confirmed. 'Futile' was on the DNACPR order on the paperwork that must have gone with him, written with reference to the chances of successful resuscitation.

We were careful and proactive in trying to avoid exactly the situation I am writing about, but it happened anyway. Unexpectedly, he had to show his documents at the border control to even higher pastures, eternity, and could not find the passport that allowed him to pass on.

(I can't help thinking about the sketches of 'stupid death' in *Horrible Histories*, with the Grim Reaper asking people at the gate of death about the reasons why they are here. In this case 'stupid cardiopulmonary resuscitation attempt' or 'stupid transfer' springs to my mind.)

In his last weeks, there were several meetings with his wife and family members. The son was closely involved – he is a community nurse and knows this field of work and decision-making very well. We talked about his father's progressive dementia and the process of slowing down, losing weight, and slowly fading away that we could see happening in front of our eyes. A while ago I investigated the weight loss with blood tests and even a CT scan of chest, abdomen, and pelvis, looking for diseases like cancer, but nothing showed up. There was also his wife. She worried a lot about him, and she was also becoming increasingly frail.

Three weeks ago, the case came again to my attention. I had a long conversation with the son, and we agreed to have a best-interest meeting outlining plans for all 'what-if' eventualities. What if there is a sudden illness and he dies? What if he develops a chest infection, should he go to hospital? The family including the son, who has power of attorney for health and finances, agreed that a natural death should be allowed to happen.

Last week the wife fell and broke her hip. She had to go to the hospital, which meant that her husband could not stay at home, so he had to be relocated to a nursing home – Higher Pastures.

And the story ends here. Our what-if scenarios did not include the possibility of the couple being separated and him needing to go independently to a nursing home. It did not include the importance of the DNACPR form needing to be visible for any new person, unfamiliar with the case.

At Border Control, the passport needs to be visible. It is not enough to just have a passport ....

Reflection

DNACPR orders occupy a central and mystical position in the conversations surrounding death and dying. The question of ceilings of investigations and treatment is a much more challenging one than the question about whether to attempt CPR – which is always futile in the context of terminal illness.[13] The conversation about issuing a DNACPR order is a figurative one, its essence being about the meaning and value of the patient's life in the symbolic order rather than a literal discussion about the likelihood of successful resurrection in the event of death.

The approach of the clinician plays a significant role in how the message is heard. Whilst there is a public outcry about doctors having issued DNACPR orders about patients without consulting them or their significant others, it is not our experience that people get upset if such a conversation takes place in the context of investment into their care and their life. In contrast, our stories highlight the dilemmas of DNACPR orders when there is rationing across all levels of care – from community to hospital, from ward to Intensive Care Unit.

Working with DNACPR forms in different contexts turns them into *boundary objects*.[14] Boundary objects are *things* with a function in everyday practice; and also meaning in the symbolic order. The form, with its white front sheet and red frame, is associated with the bureaucracy of death and dying. It is an important item in the sociomaterial context of healthcare settings, like the scriptures on an altar in a church. Only professionals of a certain rank are allowed to sign this document. Its location, access, storage, and display on patient files and in patients' homes are of paramount importance and significance. The wording on patients' records tells a lot about the position of the author. 'Patient wishes not to be resuscitated'; 'patient chooses not to be resuscitated' are common wordings. There is a belief that this document needs to be signed by the patient or by their next of kin. Of course, there is a psychological aspect to this. Does this mean the patient or their relative is signing their life away?

I remember the learning disability (LD) psychiatrist who declared during the first COVID-19 lockdown that once his frail patients were released from secondary care, their hospital DNACPR forms would not be valid in his territory, the psychiatric hospital for patients with learning disabilities. I am guessing he wanted to prove the point that in his territory, as opposed to the acute hospital, residents' lives are worth more. He did not think about the mechanics of dying and CPR and its consequences. As a matter of fact, one very ill resident experienced a traumatic death in hospital. Carers at the hospital who knew her experienced moral injury after this haunting event which occurred during the first wave of COVID-19. If the patient had been allowed to stay in the LD hospital, loving staff would have been allowed to nurse her in her dying phase and she would have remained in her familiar environment.

A trainee tells me that there is a surgeon who does not issue DNACPR forms for his patients because he believes that then they will get a substandard service. When I vehemently protest and tell him it isn't true, it only applies to medical procedures not performed *after* death, another trainee says that there is in fact some justification for the surgeon's perceptions and actions. He, the trainee, has noticed that nurses ask for help in a different manner when someone has a DNACPR order in place. 'She is end of life, take your time', he has heard. And in handovers, 'What is the diagnosis? Oh she's DNACPR'.[15]

I want to un-hear what I have just heard. I tell my patients that everything that can be done for them will be done as a matter of urgency until the point of death. And then death will be allowed to happen. 'I will do everything for you until you die but once dead, there will be no attempt to kickstart the heart in a dying body, it would not work.' I believe this to be true but now I wonder about the unintended consequences of actions taken with the best intentions.

It is very difficult to predict death, even for the experts. Only Oscar, the famous cat in a Canadian nursing home can reliably predict who is next.[16] Nevertheless, terms like 'actively dying' or 'immediate threat to life' are commonly used categories to regulate workflow. The decision-making process in the ambiguous no man's land which lies between the zone of death avoidance and the zone of death acceptance can be dramatic. This is the twilight zone which lies between two opposing camps – storming ahead with the activities of escalating diagnostic and therapeutic activities – or in contrast focusing on acceptance and controlling symptoms, regardless of their origin.

Glossary of Terms

Advance Decision to Refuse Treatment (ADRT or 'Living Will'): A legally binding, written statement in which a patient specifies which treatment they do not wish to receive in particular circumstances. Common examples are refusal to be ventilated or to be kept alive by a feeding tube in the event of terminal cancer resulting in an inability to breathe or eat independently, even if this refusal results in death. An ADRT only becomes relevant at the point when the patient loses capacity and can no longer express their own wishes. An ADRT must be witnessed, and copies given to the primary health care team and other medical professionals involved in end-of-life care. There are many websites which provide templates and guidance on writing ADRTs.

Advance Statement of Wishes: A statement expressing a patient's preferences – and may include anything from the food they are given to the care they receive. Again, it only becomes relevant when the patient can no longer express their own wishes. It is not legally binding but can be used to aid in decision-making.

Cremation Form: A form, signed by two doctors, that allows the body of a deceased person to be cremated. The doctors need to have seen and inspected the body and agree on the circumstances and mode of death.

Do Not Attempt Cardiopulmonary Resuscitation (DNACPR): A written record stating that CPR should not be attempted in the event of cardiac arrest (usually because a successful outcome is extremely unlikely). A DNACPR is a clinical decision, but it is good practice to take into consideration the views of the patient and his or her family.

Lasting Power of Attorney (LPA): An LPA can be made for either financial matters and/or for health and welfare. It is a legally binding decision which affords the nominated 'attorney' legal power to make decisions on behalf of the patient when they lose the capacity to make their own. An attorney may be able to override an ADRT if they were appointed after the ADRT was written. An application to appoint an LPA must be made when the patient is still deemed to have capacity. The relevant forms are available online and can be completed without the help of a lawyer.

Medical Certificate of Cause of Death (MCCD): After a death has been verified, a certificate (Medical Certificate of Cause of Death – MCCD) must be completed and submitted to the local registrar of births, marriages, and deaths. The certificate must be completed by a doctor who is GMC-registered with a licence to practice. In addition to other details required on the certificate, the doctor must provide a cause of death. The cause entered is a matter of clinical judgement, determined by weighing up the patient's recent and past medical history and the circumstances of their death. When a doctor cannot reasonably give a likely cause of death, the case must be submitted to the coroner for investigation which may include a post-mortem examination of the body. The patient must have been seen by a doctor within the last 28 days for a death certificate to be valid. If this is not the case, the coroner must be informed.

Treatment Escalation Plan/Care Plan: Written document outlining ceilings of treatment.

Verification of Life Extinct (aka Verification of the Fact of Death or Death Verification): Death is defined as 'irreversible loss of the capacity for consciousness, combined with the irreversible loss of capacity to breathe'. The examination includes an assessment of breathing, heart action, and cerebral action (absence of pupil reaction to light). General Medical Council (GMC) registered doctors are entitled to verify life extinct as are nurses and paramedics who have had additional mandated training. Death verification allows the body of the deceased to be removed from the place of death and brought to the chapel of rest.

Notes

1. Caitlin Doughty, *From Here to Eternity: Travelling the World to Find the Good Death* (UK: Hachette, 2017).

2. Kathryn Mannix, *Listen: How to Find the Words for Tender Conversations* (London: Harper Collins, 2021).

3. Joan Bakewell, 'We Need to Talk About Death', *BBC Radio 4*, 3 December (2017), https://www.bbc.co.uk/programmes/b083pd1p.

4. Anonymous Dominican Friar, *Ars Moriendi* (Oxford: Oxford Polonsky Foundation, Bodleian Library 1415).

5. Kathryn Mannix, *With the End in Mind: How to Live and Die Well* (Chichester: William Collins, 2018).

6. Catriona Kennedy, Patricia Brooks-Young, Carol Brunton Gray, Phil Larkin, Michael Connolly, Bodil Wilde-Larsson, Maria Larsson, Tracy Smith, and Susie Chater, 'Diagnosing Dying: An Integrative Literature Review', *BMJ Supportive & Palliative Care* 4, no. 3 (2014): 263–70.

7. Bob Spall, Sue Read, and David Chantry, 'Metaphor: Exploring Its Origins and Therapeutic Use in Death, Dying and Bereavement', *International Journal of Palliative Nursing* 7, no. 7 (2001): 345–53.

8. Charlotte Hommerberg, Anna W. Gustafsson, and Anna Sandgren, 'Battle, Journey, Imprisonment and Burden: Patterns of Metaphor Use in Blogs About Living with Advanced Cancer', *BMC Palliative Care* 19, no. 1 (2020): 1–10.

9. General Medical Council, *Ethical Guidance* (London: General Medical Guidance, 2022).

10. Julia Neuberger, C. Guthrie, and D. Aaronovitch, *More Care, Less Pathway: A Review of the Liverpool Care Pathway* (UK: Department of Health, 2013).

11. John Berger and Jean Mohr, *A Fortunate Man*, 1st ed. (Edinburgh: Canongate, 1967).

12. Caitríona Cox and Zoë Fritz, 'Presenting Complaint: Use of Language that Disempowers Patients', *BMJ* 377 (2022): e066720.

13. Stefan Timmermans, *Sudden Death and the Myth of CPR* (Philadelphia, PA: Temple University Press, 1999).

14. Susan Leigh Star and James R. Griesemer, 'Institutional Ecology, Translations' and Boundary Objects: Amateurs and Professionals in Berkeley's Museum of Vertebrate Zoology, 1907–39', *Social Studies of Science* 19, no. 3 (1989): 387–420.

15. Paul Crawford and Brian Brown, 'Fast Healthcare: Brief Communication, Traps and Opportunities', *Patient Education and Counseling* 82, no. 1 (2011): 3–10.

16. David M. Dosa, 'A Day in the Life of Oscar the Cat', *New England Journal of Medicine* 357, no. 4 (2007): 328.

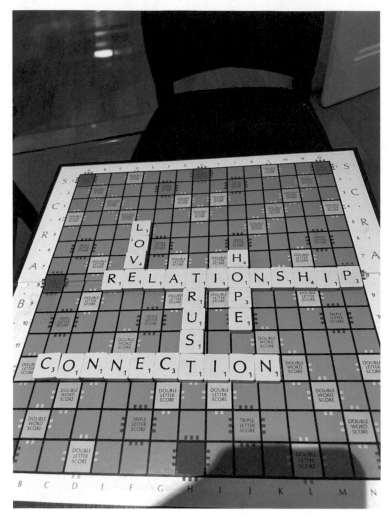

FIGURE 7.1: Scrabble 7, 'Love', Rupal Shah and Jens Foell, 2021.

7.

A Labour of Love: Why It Is That General Practice Is Still a Good Place to Work

On the Road Again - From Dusk Till Dawn: Doctoring as a Road Movie

The shift begins. A brief meeting in the office, check equipment, check documents, have a glimpse at the jobs on the screen, and see which jobs are coming up. I take the *Toughbook*, the mobile laptop with aerial connection to the central server, Adastra, meaning 'to the stars'. The *Toughbook* is logistics, patient note diary, and work planner all in one. I wonder what challenges I should expect on the job: the *Toughbook* is designed to assist special forces in their raids,to survive explosions and it has credentials for working on oil platforms and in desert conditions. On the other hand, the vehicle that is loaned to us occupies a miserable position in the prestige hierarchy of cars – a Skoda with added extras.

We have a Skoda with added extras! The extras include bright lights at each side of the car to illuminate house numbers and names; and a sign saying 'doctor' on top, which from behind reads 'meddyg', doctor in Welsh.

Off we go. The *Toughbook* heralds each new job on the system with a little *ping*. We need to organize the sequence of jobs by urgency and by geography. People may have to wait.

Mountains and sea dominate the epic scenery. Most tasks are in the limbo land of living with frailty and disability at the intersection of secondary care, primary care and end-of-life services. There is a rhythm: the encounters are intense and emotionally charged and the doctor has to bring all their resources to the job: asking the right questions at the right time in the right tone, questions to the patient and the people who made the call. Family members or others may speak for the patient and the doctor has to negotiate with them about what should be done. In Out-of-Hours, visits are away games, I am a guest, there are no hospital rules and there is no reception. During home visits, the information about the life world of the patient is almost overwhelming: too much information! Pictures on the wall, paraphernalia of living with illness and disability, media, clutter, everything matters, and everything tells a story.

The contrast is intense. Many patients' lifeworlds have shrunk to their house, a chair, or even their bed. Yet through the window, I see the majestic backdrop of Snowdonia. The conversation about what to do or not, what is wise, which battles to take on, and how to assist a good death at home or avoid death at all cost, these conversations are intense. Back in the car, I type notes in the *Toughbook*, as we head to our next destination. It is an idyll. No pop-up messaging, no people knocking at my door, no extra list with multiple decision points.No, it is a pure journey in a quiet space with a quiet driver. Bliss. Some words. We are together. Hedges, dry walls, cattle in meadows, wind-bent trees, epic views, it is a road movie. 'Stunning view! Shame it is Amlwch we are looking at', says the driver.

We become familiar with the geography and organization of supported care. Nursing homes, residential homes and dementia care. We are regulars.

Tomte Tummetot was my favourite childhood cartoon figure. In this Swedish children's book, he is the good goblin who looks after the farm at night. When our car rolls up the driveway of a former Manor House, now a Care Home, I feel like Dr. Tummetot entering the scene with his worn leather bag and doing what doctors have been doing for the last 2000 years. I visit the helpless, I come in crisis, I talk and touch. This is the essence of doctoring; it is the archetypal scene of medicine and I have to use my senses, my doctoring craft, and my human warmth. Archaic medicine. It is extremely satisfying.

When the day dawns and we are heading back to base, I feel tired and happy. Another night, some more locations are added to my mind map, and more memories are attached to places and situations.

It is a good place to work.

Bad News

I had been trying to contact Joan for the past week. A chest X-ray taken during a recent hospital admission for pneumonia revealed possible lung cancer but she self-discharged before she was told the diagnosis. She didn't have a landline and wasn't answering her mobile phone. I was walking past her tower block on my way home from the surgery, so I decided to try and tell her the news in person.

I first met Joan about fifteen years ago, soon after I started at the practice. She grew up in a poor area of Glasgow as one of seven children. She had invisible wounds from her childhood, which revealed themselves as I got to know her. It might be why she had fallen out with all her siblings over the years, except for one older brother who lived near her in London. She told me that he had always looked out for her when no one else did. She was quick to notice any real or perceived slight. Enough people had let her down in her life to make her frugal with her trust and quick to withdraw it.

Because she wasn't housebound, I had never seen her at home before. She lived on the seventh floor of a tall grey Council block. The paint was peeling from around the front entrance and when I got buzzed in, a heady mix of cannabis laced with urine hit me in the face.

The Council blocks in the Estate nearest our surgery were built in the 1970s. A patient I got to know when I first started working at the surgery told me how delighted she and her parents had been when they were rehoused in one of these flats – they were the height of modernity back then, with central heating, modern plumbing, and reliable electricity. They held the promise of a new future where their residents' lives mattered, and families could have opportunities they had been denied for generations. This is another promise that hasn't been kept. Our area is plagued with gang crime. The boys who are knifed or who are the hoodie-wearing attackers live on this Estate. The explanation that is felt but not articulated amongst our politicians is that the fault lies with the people who live here, whom they blame for not being able to offer their children a brighter future.

But how would you go about that if it were you?

There are different lifts for odd-numbered floors and for even. But in any case, on that day neither lift was working and so I took the stairs, feeling a cold draft on my face as I climbed up. It was getting dark and I wished that I didn't feel on edge as I made my way upstairs. When I passed a young Black man running downstairs, I flinched and my pulse raced. My reaction disappointed me.

Joan opened the door cautiously, with the chain done up and was clearly astonished to see me.

'Oh my God, it's bad news isn't it?', she said as she let me in.

I sat with her in the front room recovering my breath. We were still for a few moments, and neither of us said anything. I took in her front room, the worn sofa, covered in a colourful-knitted blanket and magazines, the single armchair, and the television which she switched off when I sat down. We looked at one another and it seemed brutal to break the silence and end that moment. 'Joan, I don't know, but I'm afraid it might be – I'm so sorry.' I told her about the diagnosis. I was expecting tears and distress, but actually she was surprisingly calm.

'You know, I'm not surprised. I thought it would be that, I knew all along really, it's why I couldn't stay in that hospital any longer. Well, I'm just glad it was you who told me.'

There was a moment when both of us had our guards down. We could acknowledge that life can deal you these curve balls. I couldn't help her to dodge it, all I could do was stand next to her when it came spinning towards her. 'Well I'm just glad it was you who told me.' Those words kept echoing in my head for a long time afterwards, bringing tears to my eyes unexpectedly. The privilege of being allowed to stand next to her, being part of each other's stories, those moments of connection that dissolve me, that pull the best bits of me out of me, that's why I want to keep working as a GP.

The Leather Strap
Sociomateriality, Sustainability, Procurement

What is this?

An arcane torture device? A corrective chair for naughty children?

What is the purpose of this device?

This well-worn apparatus is an Oswestry stand. It is used in the rehabilitation of people for whom standing up is a challenge

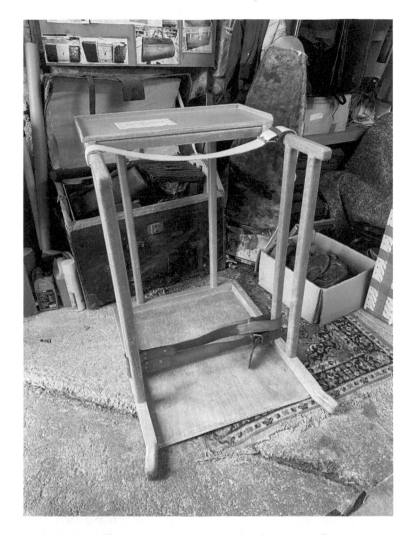

FIGURE 7.2: The contraption (Oswestry stand). Jens Foell, 2020.

because they need support to stabilize their body against the forces of gravity. Therefore, there are scaffolding wooden braces and a table to grasp. Flexible leather straps stabilize the legs and prevent them from collapsing. This device provides a semi-flexible scaffold for bodies in need of support to maintain a vertical posture.

It has long been popular with patients and staff in the physiotherapy department. You can see the traces of contact with wheelchairs at the widening entry beams. The surfaces are worn.

Then one leather belt snapped after years of wear and tear. The belts at the bottom show how they have been used over time.

As it is impossible to get a new leather strap for this outdated apparatus from the official NHS supply chain, the device has been earmarked for the scrap heap.

But the Physiotherapist knows a craftsman who specializes in repairing antique leather goods. He repairs Georgian gun cases, aristocratic crocodile leather vanity boxes, art deco watches – and now the Oswestry stand. He does not charge for this repair. Without this improvisation and generosity, the apparatus would have ended up on one of the scrap heaps at the rear end of the hospital.

The Physiotherapist breached orders. She did the right thing, and she did not do things right. There are rules and regulations for procurement and repair. Bringing a device to an antique repair shop sits firmly outside these rules and regulations.

But without these micro-breaches and acts of generosity, the NHS would not function. At the same time, they deviate from the rule book and should not exist.

In my personal experience, crutches and similar assistive devices are objects that invite the absurdity of bureaucracy. Think back to the chapter 'Weaponized Bureaucracy', 'Life Is Xerox'. Another illustration is a patient I recently came across, an otherwise fit and healthy but hypermobile PhD student (in Sports Science) with acute sciatica. The pain and weakness were so severe that she could not get up and walk from bed to toilet. She did not want to waste NHS resources. She did not want to call an ambulance or get admitted. She wanted to stay at home and allow nature to heal her sciatica, but she urgently needed crutches. The task to organize this fell on me, the visiting GP.

As a GP I don't have access to crutches. I was not aware of how difficult it can be to get a simple device that enables the patient to offload the painful region and hopefully use fewer drugs. The Physiotherapist at the local hospital said they would not give crutches to anyone without first assessing them and taking measurements. 'The patient needs to be seen', she said. I replied, 'But that's exactly the problem, she cannot even go two metres from bed to toilet! And she does not NEED to be seen!' I failed to get anywhere. The Physiotherapist suggested community services. Community services asked for a referral and said they could deal with matters hopefully within the next two weeks.

At this point, I gave up and called someone I know on another ward, where I had previously noticed a selection of crutches. I collected a pair and delivered them to the student. It is yet again an example of a personal relationship mitigating broader (dysfunctional) exchanges based on a protocol that does not allow discretion. On the ground level, these relationships of give and take, micro-trust and mutual support make things happen that otherwise get blocked in the organizational bureaucracy where the Computer says 'No'.

Labour of Love

Prydain ward is like a sanctuary for me. This sanctuary caters for people who would otherwise find it very, very difficult to find a nurturing place in life. They have profound learning disabilities, and their impairments are deemed too complex and too difficult for any service to meet their needs in 'normal' community settings. Administratively, Prydain belongs to the Mental Health hospital. The patients are inpatients. Every breath they take, every move they make is meticulously captured in written files.

Many of these residents have spent all their lives in institutions. This ward is officially an interim placement for people with severe complex needs, but some have stayed there for years and years.

As the local GP, I visit the ward once a week to look after the residents there – primary care services are contracted to deal with the 'other' that is beyond the scope of psychiatrists. What exactly this 'other' is, remains to be seen, and will probably never be clearly defined and demarcated.

For me, there is another 'other'. I am called on to make impossible judgments. Many of the predicaments are impossible to address. 'He is not his usual self' is often the curtain raiser and my job is to ascertain whether this could be due to a so far unnoticed illness, or disease progression, or random variations in being present in the world or simply an off-day or bad mood. The residents have profound disabilities and often cannot articulate

195

their distress. I rely heavily on the observations of the staff looking after them. I can feel that they are attached to the residents. They speak about their patients like mothers about the children they worry about. I am convinced that without this love many of the residents would have died years ago. Some are very frail and very old, and they have statistically outlived their grim life expectancy. Something is going right here.

Goronwy is one of the figureheads of Prydain ward. Everybody knows Gron. He smokes a pipe, he knows what he wants, he does his thing, and he has spent many years of his life on this ward. This ward is his Hotel California, where he checked in and never left. Then, over the course of months, he developed abdominal problems and eventually jaundice. He was all yellow. Something was clearly not right, and the reason turned out to be a blockage of his bile duct from cancer. He needed to go to the District General Hospital. There was a bitter row between the hospital and Prydain ward about their respective dominance in his care, about his 'safety'. Eventually, the ward staff won and Gron was allowed to go back home, where everybody knows him, where he can have his little escapes and smoke his pipe in a corner underneath the 'No Smoking' sign.

I have never seen such care for the dying. Gardeners performed loops of honour on the lawn next to Prydain ward. Staff cooked his favourite food. We had best-interest-meetings and the last days of his life were an ongoing celebration of his life. I have never seen anything like this, even in private institutions for privileged members of society in London.

Even the local Funeral Director wrote,

> I would just like to send you a message acknowledging the obvious care and love you and your team showed to Goronwy before and after we were called to Prydain, after his passing. In the 30 plus years I have been responding to call outs, this was one of the rare occasions when my colleague and I remarked on the time, care and effort that had been given to getting Gron ready for his final journey, and the staff on duty even at that late hour were all present and gave him a guard of honour – a truly lovely touch.

8.
Final Reflection – Image Reviewing

The idealized GP still lurks in our collective imaginations[1] – the archetypal, community-based doctor who operates in a low-tech or no-tech environment as an independent craftsman, enjoying a relationship of perfect trust and patriarchal benevolence. Although this vision is specious, only generated by donning a metaphorical pair of rose-tinted glasses, hospital colleagues may nevertheless have such a figure in mind when they formulate their letters with instructions for the GP.

Sociologist David Armstrong portrayed the struggle for power in healthcare as a competition for control over uncertainty.[2] The archetypal GP no longer dominates this space of uncertainty – other voices have emerged. The voices of previously neglected, oppressed, and marginalized groups have risen, often against resistance; and the stale, male, pale bearer of authority and social control is being actively challenged, progressively more so since the 1960s.[2,3,4] A combination of developments have changed the power dynamics in healthcare – industrialization, standardized evaluation, commodification, and increased regulation.[5,6] The medical profession has had to re-evaluate its position in the field,[7] as the 'E' in EBM changed its meaning and *eminence*-based medicine gave way to *evidence*-based medicine in the 1990s.[8,9,10] Primary care is characterized by tolerating uncertainty with regard to clinical decision-making, an idea which is encompassed in GP descriptions of professionalism. Yet the space of uncertainty is now dominated by processes which aim for certainty.[11]

This power shift gave prominence to the emerging class of managers. The requirements of industrialized medicine to base itself on measurable quality standards have had parallel developments in the increasing bureaucratization of care and, more recently, the digitalization of care.[10,12] All these processes are predicated on the reduction of complexity.[13] They aim to break complex situations down into simple binary steps, whether for the purpose of coding (for programmes and platforms), research protocols, guidelines, or organizational protocols.

In *2001: A Space Odyssey*, Stanley Kubrick highlights the shift of power from human agent to IT, personified by a **h**euristically programmed **al**gorithmic (HAL) computer, the sentient computer programme assisting the space mission.[14] It depicts the power clash between human operator, IT programme and ultimately the organizations and forces who programmed this digital interface. In a seminal scene, Astronaut Bowman asks to enter the spaceship, but the former assistant HAL turns the tables:

BOWMAN:	Open the pod door, Hal.
BOWMAN:	Open the pod bay doors please, Hal. Open the pod bay doors please, Hal. Hello, Hal, do you read me? Hello, Hal, do you read me? Do you read me, Hal? Do you read me, Hal? Hello, Hal, do you read me? Hello, Hal, do you read me? Do you read me, Hal?
HAL:	Affirmative, Dave. I read you.
BOWMAN:	Open the pod bay doors, Hal.
HAL:	I'm sorry, Dave. I'm afraid I can't do that.
BOWMAN:	What's the problem?
HAL:	I think you know what the problem is just as well as I do.
BOWMAN:	What are you talking about, Hal?
HAL:	This mission is too important for me to allow you to jeopardise it.
BOWMAN:	I don't know what you're talking about, Hal.
HAL:	I know that you and Frank were planning to disconnect me. And I'm afraid that's something I cannot allow to happen.
BOWMAN:	Where the hell did you get that idea, Hal?
HAL:	Dave! Although you took very thorough precautions in the pod against my hearing you, I could see your lips move.
BOWMAN:	Alright, Hal. I'll go in through the emergency airlock.

HAL:	Without your space helmet, Dave, you're going to find that rather difficult.
BOWMAN:	Hal, I won't argue with you anymore. Open the doors.
HAL:	Dave, this conversation can serve no purpose anymore. Goodbye.
BOWMAN:	Hal. Hal. Hal. Hal. Hal.

The computer said 'No'.

Within the context of primary care, the stereotypical, archetypal GP practised reactive medicine and responded to crises, with little challenge to his autonomy and authority. The doctor portrayed in the Rockwell painting 'Doctor and the Doll' represents the archetype. He sits in a comfortable leather armchair and the certificate displayed prominently on his wooden cabinet is proof of his membership of the guild of doctors, credentials underscoring his craftsmanship, his eminence. The nature of primary care has changed beyond recognition since this painting was created in the interwar years. As Tudor-Hart and Armstrong point out, the role of the GP has dramatically expanded, incorporating the tasks of large-scale, standardized surveillance, and preventative medicine.[15,16]

Contemporary medicine encapsulates competing principles of production – industrialized care and craftsmanship. The principle of industrialization relies on breaking down complex production processes and delegating simple tasks to lower-paid people who do not have control over their product or their workload. In contrast, the craftsmanship paradigm places the worker in a position of ownership and autonomy – and gives them pride in the product.[17,18] To a certain degree, medicine is a craft. In this view, it incorporates knowledge, emotional engagement, and wisdom.[19,20] It cannot be broken down into reproducible smaller steps. Primary care ideology emphasizes these aspects by calling the work of GPs 'holistic' and assuming that the whole is bigger than the sum of the parts.[21,22] It implies that the work of the GP CANNOT be carried out by a succession of rules. It includes the human element, years of practice, imagination, and emotional availability. These are the ingredients needed to create and sustain relationships. Only the GP as a generalist has the skills to examine the whole body, regardless of the age of the patient, and to prescribe across the boundaries of body and mind.

On the other hand, the simple administration of surveillance medicine, preventative polypharmacy, and the regulation of access and timings demands sophisticated sets of rules to steer the flow of tasks. The contemporary version of the archetype can only be imagined in conjunction with a call centre, complete with mobile phones and computer terminals. All these interfaces have an influence on the way information is communicated, captured, modulated, and processed. As in a Hadron collider, these information particles have their own life and leave traces. Each mini-dilemma requires hierarchical legitimation when determining resource allocation in primary care and NHS 111 or 999 call centres.

Being rooted in a paradigm of control, the spin-offs create unanswered questions, micro-dilemmas, and ethical dilemmas – borderline abnormal blood results, iatrogenesis, faulty communication, and care pathways all shrouded in a cloak of anonymity. In a way, the rules of order create disorder and have unforeseen consequences. The micro-dilemmas need closure, which requires administrative processes to come up with solutions, calling into play hierarchies, systems, and processes, such as multidisciplinary team meetings or best-interest meetings. The primary healthcare environment has become more fragmented, with more part-time players and a more limited scope of expertise. Contemporary primary care demonstrates that it is possible to break the mystery of 'undifferentiated primary care' down into a composition of sub-delegated tasks, but in parallel, it raises the challenge of how these tasks are coherently combined.[23] The desire for simplification has brought with it a wealth of bureaucratization, requiring new training, new mandates, and new risk assessments, all of which take on a life of their own and generate roadblocks for service users, i.e., patients.

Notes

1. Mary Winkler, 'Doctor and Doll', *AMA Journal of Ethics* 4, no. 2 (2002): 41–44.

2. David Armstrong, 'Professionalism, Indeterminacy and the EBM Project', *BioSocieties* 2, no. 1 (2007): 73–84.

3. E. Shorter, 'History of the Doctor-Patient-Relationship', in *Companion Encyclopedia of the History of Medicine*, eds. R. Porter and W. Bynum (London: Routledge, 1993).

4. David Armstrong, 'Actors, Patients and Agency: A Recent History', *Sociology of Health & Illness* 36, no. 2 (2014): 163–74.

5. Avedis Donabedian, 'Evaluating the Quality of Medical Care', *The Milbank Memorial Fund Quarterly* 44, no. 3 (1966): 166–206.

6. G. Scambler, 'Liberty's Command: Liberal Ideology, the Mixed Economy and the British Welfare State', in *Mind, State and Society: Social History of Psychiatry and Mental Health in Britain 1960–2010*, eds. N. Bouras and G. Ikkos (Cambridge: Cambridge University Press, 2021).

7. Working Party of the Royal College of Physicians, 'Doctors in Society. Medical Professionalism in a Changing World', *Clinical Medicine (London, England)* 5, no. 6 Suppl 1 (2005): S5–S40.

8. Trisha Greenhalgh, Jeremy Howick, and Neal Maskrey, 'Evidence-Based Medicine: A Movement in Crisis', *BMJ* 348 (2014): g3725.

9. Mark Tonelli, 'The Philosophical Limits of Evidence-Based Medicine', *Academic Medicine* 73 (1998): 1234–40.

10. David L. Sackett, M. C. Rosenberg William, J. A. Muir Gray, R. Brian Haynes, and W. Scott Richardson, *Evidence-Based Medicine: What It Is and What It Isn't* (UK: British Medical Journal Publishing Group, 1996), 71–72.

11. Rupal Shah, Sanjiv Ahluwalia, and John Spicer, 'A Crisis of Identity: What Is the Essence of General Practice', *British Journal of General Practice* 71 (2021): 246–47.

12. Haridimos Tsoukas and Mary Jo Hatch, 'Complex Thinking, Complex Practice: The Case for a Narrative Approach to Organizational Complexity', *Human Relations* 54, no. 8 (2001): 979–1013.

13. Frederic W. Hafferty and Dana Levinson, 'Moving Beyond Nostalgia and Motives: Towards a Complexity Science View of Medical Professionalism', *Perspectives in Biology and Medicine* 51, no. 4 (2008): 599–615.

14. Stanley Kubrick, *2001: A Space Odyssey* (1968).

15. David Armstrong, 'The Rise of Surveillance Medicine', *Sociology of Health & Illness* 17, no. 3 (1995): 393–404.

16. Julian Tudor Hart, *The Political Economy of Health Care: A Clinical Perspective* (Bristol: Policy Press, 2006).

17. Richard Sennett, *The Craftsman* (London: Yale University Press, 2008).

18. Jochem Kroezen, Davide Ravasi, Innan Sasaki, Monika Żebrowska, and Roy Suddaby, 'Configurations of Craft: Alternative Models for Organizing Work', *Academy of Management Annals* 15, no. 2 (2021): 502–36.

19. Fredrik Svenaeus, 'Hermeneutics of Medicine in the Wake of Gadamer: The Issue of Phronesis', *Theoretical Medicine and Bioethics* 24, no. 5 (2003): 407–31.

20. Roger Kneebone, *Expert: Understanding the Path to Mastery* (UK: Penguin, 2020).

21. Joshua Freeman, 'Towards a Definition of Holism', *British Journal of General Practice* 55, no. 511 (2005): 154–55.

22. Kath Checkland, Stephen Harrison, Ruth McDonald, Suzanne Grant, Stephen Campbell, and Bruce Guthrie, 'Biomedicine, Holism and General Medical Practice: Responses to the 2004 General Practitioner Contract', *Sociology of Health & Illness* 30, no. 5 (2008): 788–803.

23. J. Mohan, 'Post-Fordism and Welfare: An Analysis of Change in the British Health Sector', *Environment and Planning A* 27, no. 10 (1995): 1555–76.

Conclusion

You feel like the GP is a machine which is processing you.
(Rupal's father-in-law, August 2021)

Patient-centred, personalized care is the mantra of the National Health Service (NHS).[1] In its constitution, the NHS speaks directly to the citizen patient and pledges to 'put you, your family and carers at the centre of decisions that affect you or them'.[2] However, the health system is designed with population health in mind, rather than relational, individualized care. This creates a paradox, which GPs and other primary care clinicians are left to negotiate. Clinicians are charged with daily decisions about rationing, incentivized for adding people to chronic disease registers (and taking them off) and in salesman mode, persuading people to take medications to delay or prevent expensive, catastrophic events such as heart attacks and strokes; or batting away requests for referrals which do not fit with local guidance. This population health approach has benefits but does not fit naturally with a personalized care paradigm. It is therefore an implicit but fundamental part of the job of the primary care clinician to navigate a path of individualized care that is set against a backdrop of standardization – to negotiate the tension between the patient as representing a population average (as in research and policy) and the patient as an individual, whose life circumstances have to be taken into account. In this way, GPs and other primary care clinicians serve two masters who have different priorities and value systems. Contemporary semi-automated healthcare thus conceptualizes GPs as street-level bureaucrats who must constantly negotiate the needs of the client with the agenda of the organization.[3]

Bureaucracy can lead to cynicism, boundaried working, and disengagement, but it can also be used as a lever to achieve societal change and improvements to population health – an example is the COVID-19 vaccination programme, which could be rolled out efficiently because of the detailed health records held within General Practice. Data provides hard evidence of inequalities in healthcare and is thus a lever which can be used to force political change. The tension arises because protocols, algorithms, and guidelines are by their nature generic; their purpose being to remove uncertainty and variability, to improve population health outcomes, and to reduce the reputational risk faced by healthcare institutions. Unfortunately, this can be at the expense of considering the wider, societal effects of industrialized care.[4] It is also at odds with the mission statement of person-centred care and with the reality of clinical practice, which requires the clinician to respond to the unique and unpredictable context of each individual patient and family, where lives are inter-connected, experience is subjective, and there are few absolute truths or certainties.[5,6]

There is therefore a disconnect between the purpose of general practice as conceptualized within the bureaucratic paradigm, the mantra of person-centred care and the lived experience of clinicians and patients.[7] The standardization of therapeutic interactions has been a consequence of the bureaucratic paradigm, where the role of the primary care clinician is to categorize and then select a pathway. A system in which protocol and algorithm govern clinical decision-making has inadvertent consequences on the mindset of clinicians, making them risk-averse and reluctant to venture into the complexity of narrative and context. It may also lead to burnout since in our experience, the joy of work largely emanates from personal relationships.

General practice is facing a crisis of identity. Speaking as GPs ourselves, we propose that we need to decide what gives meaning to our profession and whether we are permitted to give relational, individualized care with all the messiness and uncertainty this involves and to go the extra mile; or to stick to standardization, enacting rules enshrined in protocol.[8]

There is a discretionary space in which primary care clinicians can make choices about how to enact the bureaucratic processes which structure the health service. There are multiple influences on this space. On one hand, there is bureaucracy itself, encompassing regulation, defensive medicine, boundaries, and standardization (and in the end, income and organizational reputation). On the other hand, there is individual connection, duty, nuance, discretion, context, and narrative. High-quality bureaucracy serves a useful, even essential purpose, but it should not be the only influence within the discretionary space.

It is not just medicine which faces these existential but unvoiced questions. Similar choices – craft vs. industrialization; generic vs. individualized approaches; bureaucratic vs. relational care – exist for society in general, and are particularly evident in other public service sectors, such as education, the police force, and social services.

It is beyond the scope of this book to propose detailed changes to the organization of UK primary care, but we conclude with a few thoughts on what might change the nature of this discretionary space for clinicians and thereby alter the experience of patients who access primary care.

Continuity of Care

There is incontrovertible evidence that continuity of care with a regular GP and the quality of the therapeutic alliance improves clinical outcomes (including mortality), reduces A&E attendance, and increases patient satisfaction with health services.[9,10] This approach is cost-effective too because investigations are less likely to be repeated and referrals made more judiciously, taking the context and preferences of the patient into account. Longitudinal relationships make it more probable that there is a personal connection which changes the clinician's approach, making them more willing to authentically engage with their patient, rather than retreating behind the anonymity of the medical establishment. Something which is not obvious is that it is the small, low-stake encounters (minor infections and injuries, contraception checks, etc.) that build up stores of trust and goodwill for when things get hard – this is not accounted for by the 'GP consultant' model, in which minor illness is delegated to other professionals such as nurse practitioners and physician's associates.

Continuity has to be reconciled with the fact that the majority of primary care clinicians do not work clinically five days a week and do not routinely do Out-of-Hours shifts. As we said at the start of the book, we do not advocate a return to the days when GPs were responsible for their registered patients 24 hours a day, seven days a week – times have changed so that it would be impossible to recruit enough clinicians prepared to work in this way. The reality is that there are boundaries to the care we are prepared to give, sometimes influenced by the nature of the relationships we have with particular patients (see 'Weaponized Bureaucracy').

205

Continuity – to an extent anyway – can still be possible when working part-time in big, multidisciplinary teams. Some large surgeries have been divided into much smaller, micro teams, with representation from GPs (matched for their working patterns so that one doctor from the team is available every day), nurses, healthcare assistants, and other allied health professionals such as pharmacists. Patients are allocated to a particular team so that they tend to see the same group of clinicians each time. Within this model, there should be dedicated time for teams to discuss patients they have seen, ask each other questions, and fill in narrative gaps with the help of colleagues. In effect, it is like trying to divide the supermarket up into smaller, inter-connected corner shops.

Many practices already operate systems that facilitate continuity of care for the ones who benefit most from it: for example, patients with frailty, multimorbidity, and severe mental health problems. This is when intensive primary care matters most and knowing the patient makes a huge difference, so patients within these disease registers often have a named doctor. It is the opposite to 'taxi-rank-medicine' or 'Uber-medicine' as Jeremy Hunt, Chair of the Health and Social Care Select Committee, termed it in 2022.[11]

Prioritizing continuity values and encourages human engagement and a humanist approach to healthcare. But as things stand, continuity of care does not formally feature in any of the national performative schemes, whereby practices are financially incentivized to achieve particular clinical outcomes. The 2023/24 NHS England access targets are likely to make things worse, not better as far as continuity goes, with pressure on practices to assign incoming patient requests to any available clinician to deal with as soon as possible. Continuity has also not made it to the Care Quality Commission's (CQC) checklist. Unfortunately, our regulatory system feeds into and inadvertently encourages an impersonal, tick-box approach, which privileges measurable outputs over relationships. There is a missed opportunity to anchor the human dimension of care within systems of governance and reimbursement.

Control and Connection
Training and then practising in a culture which is dominated by one-size-fits-all rules, regulations, templates, and algorithms has the effect of altering the nature of the interaction between patients and clinicians and between team members. Other authors have

described the effect that controls mechanisms such as surveillance and monitoring have on the way in which members of any institution relate to one another and to clients.[3] It encourages defensive practice and a target-driven culture, the pitfalls of which have been highlighted time and again in reports about NHS failings (e.g., North Staffordshire 2009, Telford Maternity 2003–2022). Healthcare systems may have failed to mobilize an important resource by not nurturing the intrinsic motivations and values of clinicians ('professionalism') and instead attempting to control behaviour by establishing external incentives and control systems.[12] As Rosenbaum says, 'The more requirements we pile on in the pursuit of being better, the less room clinicians have to determine – with their patients – what "better" really means'.[13]

Like Hercules battling the heads of Hydra, pursuing each individual incentive scheme generates additional streams of work. For example, a recent local target in England was to screen and then treat people with undiagnosed high blood pressure. For a number of patients, this will have meant starting new medications, which require regular monitoring to ensure that they are effective and are not adversely affecting kidney function. It takes time and uses up appointments. In Rupal's practice of 14,500 patients, about 400 texts are sent per month inviting patients to the surgery for some form of screening or chronic disease surveillance intervention. The effect of this and of the other incentive schemes in operation is that some people are harangued by text messages and letters into coming into the surgery, whereas others who don't fall into chronic disease categories struggle to be seen at all. The GP is becoming a nuisance cold caller, because there isn't an overview taken by policymakers about how each new target fits into the others already in existence. We are adding to the treatment burden and over-medicalization that are becoming serious problems facing society at large. There is a tipping point beyond which preventative medicine might be doing more harm than good. A syndemic framework (see 'Guidelines, Tramlines, Mindlines') that recognises and moves to address the effects of social and environmental drivers on chronic disease may be a more sustainable approach to population health than one which waits for people to become ill and then relies mostly on medical interventions. True prevention would involve tackling the social determinants of health before they manifest as chronic physical and mental disease.

Another consideration is that too much control (in the form of targets and checklists) can kill off curiosity and create a tick-box mindset, in which questions are only asked for the purpose of completing the template and gathering 'useful' information. Where there is no connection, there is no willingness to engage on an emotional level. The consultation becomes mechanistic, generic, and boundaried. The patient becomes a problem to be solved and then discarded.

Interestingly, Scotland has taken a different, less prescriptive approach to the organization of primary healthcare, with the removal of the GP quality and outcome framework (QoF) from the Scottish GP contract in 2016. QoF consists of 68 generic achievement measures across clinical, public health, and quality improvement domains and is the source of the yellow triangles that we have alluded to in previous chapters. High achievement in QoF is a quality marker as well as attracting significant financial rewards for practices. It makes up a significant percentage of the workload of GPs in England, Wales, and Northern Ireland. Removing QoF was an explicit attempt to move general practice away from an 'industrialised, biomedical, single disease focused model of care'[14] to one that could be more value-based and responsive to the local context.[15] GPs working collaboratively in 'clusters' are now asked to implement quality improvement activities which are based on the needs of their local populations. It is not yet clear what effect this will have on long-term population health or on the culture of general practice. However, there is a growing movement towards engaging and empowering communities to make strategic decisions about their health in partnership with healthcare professionals, rather than the historic top-down approach.[16]

Emotional Engagement

> Those who are unhappy have no need for anything in this world but people capable of giving them their attention. The capacity to give one's attention to a sufferer is a very rare and difficult thing; it is almost a miracle; it is a miracle. Nearly all those who think they have this capacity do not possess it. Warmth of heart, impulsiveness, pity are not enough.
>
> (Weil 2003)[17]

The focused attention that Weil describes naturally produces an emotional response in the listener. There is ambivalence within the medical establishment about the extent to which doctors should show or even feel emotion. The ideal of professional detachment is entrenched within the culture of medicine and has been ever since the invention of diagnostic instruments and tests, which shifted medicine from being an art to being a science; and thus reduced the weight given to narrative, while elevating the importance of technical interpretation.[18] Medical students are actively encouraged to maintain distance between themselves and their patients and this sends out confusingly mixed messages ('be compassionate but don't allow yourself to feel').[19] I am often asked the question by trainees, 'Is it ok to cry in front of a patient?' The worry is that, like Dr. Eskell in *A Fortunate Man*, too much emotional engagement could lead to burnout and a blurring of professional boundaries.[20] This may be true if taken to extremes. However, there are also dangers associated with ignoring emotion and with the culture of invulnerability that exists in medicine. In fact, there is evidence that not acknowledging the feelings aroused by painful, difficult encounters leads to cynicism, depression, and professional attrition.[21] Relational care brings the joy of human connection to work. It involves allowing oneself to become part of someone else's story and might actually help clinicians to flourish.[22]

As a profession, GPs should consider the effect of emotionally boundaried working and address it during training. Curiosity, compassion, and emotional engagement are key dispositions to be encouraged and rewarded. The training curriculum, embracing intelligent kindness and cultures of care, should move towards different methods of assessment which engage with the thought processes and emotional responses of trainees; and encourage critical thinking and awareness of the different influences on their practice.[23] The 'sort, fix, or send' paradigm should be challenged, with more validation given to the therapeutic benefits of listening closely and bearing witness to somebody's suffering – the 'holding work' which we have talked about throughout this book.[24,25] Paying attention to somebody else inevitably generates intimacy and vulnerability, which as a profession, GPs tend to be taught to avoid and be suspicious of; yet without them, much of what we do is meaningless for us and for our patients.

Patient satisfaction questionnaires are a mandatory part of the evidence which GPs must present for revalidation. If the format of these questionnaires were different, maybe the priorities of the consultation would change too. The Consultation and Relational

I. Please rate the following statements about today's consultation. Please tick one box for each statement and answer every statement.						
How was the doctor at...	Poor	Fair	Good	Very good	Excellent	Does not apply
1) Making you feel at ease... (being friendly and warm toward you, treating you with respect; not cold or abrupt)						
2) Letting you tell your "story"... (giving you time to fully describe your illness in your own words; not interrupting or diverting you)						
3) Really listening... (paying close attention to what you were saying; not looking at the notes or computer as you were talking)						
4) Being interested in you as a whole person... (asking/knowing relevant details about your life, your situation; not treating you as just a number)						
5) Fully understanding your concerns... (communicating that he/she had accurately understood your concerns; not overlooking or dismissing anything)						
6) Showing care and compassion... (seeming genuinely concerned, connecting with you on a human level; not being indifferent or "detached")						
7) Being positive... (having a positive approach and a positive attitude; being honest but not negative about your problems)						
8) Explaining things clearly... (fully answering your questions, explaining clearly, giving you adequate information; not being vague)						
9) Helping you to take control... (exploring with you what you can do to improve your health yourself; encouraging rather than "lecturing" you)						
10) Making a plan of action with you... (discussing the options, involving you in decisions as much as you want to be involved; not ignoring your views)						

Figure C.1: CARE measure.

Empathy CARE measure developed by Stewart Mercer and colleagues in Glasgow during the 2000s is an example of a measure of quality of care that attempts to capture connection and rapport – facets of the consultation which are not usually assessed.[26]

Risk

Many of the algorithms and protocols in existence today were designed with risk reduction in mind. The point is that reducing risk in one way usually increases it in another way. COVID-19 has taught us a lot about the complexity of risk reduction – the lockdown-generated reduction in COVID-19-related mortality increased other risks, e.g. mental health problems, bankruptcy, isolation, domestic violence, and a widening of pre-existing social inequality which meant that some families thrived whilst others sank.[27]

Similarly, patient safety is not always helpful when used as the ultimate 'check-mate'. We usually mean safety from death – possibly. However, increased investigations, referrals, and medicalization confer their own risks as does a rigid adherence to protocol. In her report to the Parliamentary Committee (2022), Joanne Reeve proposed that treatment burden will soon outstrip multimorbidity as the biggest challenge faced by patients and clinicians.[28] As Reeve points out, for the healthcare system to be functional, GPs and other clinicians need to feel they have permission to use their clinical or ethical judgement to override the protocol when needed, instead of being enslaved by it.

During the COVID-19 pandemic, an 82-year-old woman, Mrs. Z is admitted to hospital with a stroke. Unfortunately, she becomes increasingly distressed and confused during her hospital stay. She is on a surgical ward as there are no beds on the stroke unit. The hospital policy is to allow only one named visitor per patient – in this case, it is Mrs. Z's son who lives nearer to the hospital than other family members. However, his work commitments mean he can't visit every day. Mrs. Z has a very close relationship with her granddaughter, who drives for two hours to see her when she hears Mrs. Z's condition is deteriorating. She brings a fish tagine, a dish which Mrs. Z used to make for her when she was growing up. The granddaughter has done a lateral flow test which is negative. The nurse in charge refuses her admission, as it is against the rules to let her in. It is also against the rules to give Mrs. Z the food her granddaughter prepared for her. Mrs. Z dies in hospital without having been able to say goodbye to her granddaughter.

Perhaps another nurse would have chosen differently. But it is unrealistic to expect individuals who are overburdened and underpaid to make decisions which result in them shouldering extra risk and which might result in punishment.

Eraut encapsulates the problem: 'routines tend to become increasingly dysfunctional over time: not only do they fail to adjust to new circumstances but "shortcuts" gradually intrude, some of which help professionals to cope with pressure at the expense of helping their clients'.[29] The moral injury which results from having to continually act in a way that is counter to one's values and to the particularities of the context almost certainly drives burnout and attrition in a service which is already over-stretched.

There should be a level of discretion and flexibility built into the system, based on trust, whereby staff are able to act against guidelines after discussion with colleagues when the consensus is that it is justified to do so. The paradox is that trust is fundamental to good governance, but trust and control mechanisms such as protocol are uneasy bedfellows. However, despite this tension, the co-existence of trust and control are hallmarks of the predicament of a practising clinician in general practice. GPs are simultaneously patients' advocates and disciplinarians; appraisers coach their appraisees in the pursuit of a better work-life balance whilst also checking their performance on behalf of the General Medical Council (GMC). This double-bind situation is at the heart of street-level bureaucracy.

Time and Grind

A factory with an endlessly turning conveyor belt captures something of the atmosphere of general practice. Historically, GP consultations were between five and ten minutes long, although these days most GPs allow at least ten minutes per consultation. This model is outdated. It belongs to the era of the archetypal GP who had nobody to answer to, little that needed to be recorded and very few if any surveillance and monitoring requirements to meet. It is also predicated on follow-up being easy and practical – 'come and see me next week and let's talk through your other problems'. The chances of patients being able to make an appointment with the same GP on a regular basis are small unless they become poppets who are helped through the healthcare parkour by clinicians. It is not possible to simultaneously meet the ever-increasing demands of surveillance medicine and also listen attentively to a patient, make thoughtful decisions, and uncover meaning in ten minutes. 'One problem per consultation' doesn't make sense either, because problems don't exist in isolation – they are linked to past experience, social context, values, and outlook.

A ten-minute consultation is adequate for a generic, transactional, biomedical interaction or if it is one of an unfolding series of encounters which take place over a period of time. GP consultations need to be longer, but with the caveat that the extra time should be spent trying to understand the wider context of the patient and what matters to them. In the long run, this might be more efficient in terms of both time and money than short, rushed interactions, where the doctor's main agenda is to avoid running late.

Remote Consultations

In 2020, Matt Hancock who was then Secretary of State for Health and Social Care proclaimed that 'All [GP] consultations should be tele-consultations' and warned us against 'falling back into old habits', but instead advised that clinicians should be freed up to concentrate on 'what really matters'.[30] There was a public backlash against remote consulting in 2021, ironically spearheaded by the right-wing newspaper, the *Daily Mail*, which resulted in significant reputational damage to General Practice.

Remote consultations are eminently suitable for the transactional but struggle to meet the needs of patients for whom medical categorization is inadequate, whose symptoms arise at the interface of body, mind, and environment, and for whom a therapeutic approach depends upon establishing a longitudinal relationship based on mutual trust.

Generally, remote consultations in NHS primary care work better for people with the ability and confidence to express themselves in English and who have access to the right technology. Distinguishing between what can and cannot be effectively (and therefore efficiently) managed remotely is a key question for primary care, one which it is imperative to answer, in order to prevent widening disparities in access to good quality healthcare. The most pragmatic solution might be to simply let patients choose whether they want a remote or in-person appointment.

Access and the Digital Divide

Systems which rely on patients to be able to explain their symptoms accurately on an online form and to follow a flowchart of questions are cumbersome and discriminatory, making services more accessible for some than for others. The combination of multimorbidity, chronic pain, and mental health problems has a social gradient. As the Bible says, 'the poor will always be with you', but digital exclusion removes the voice of the disenfranchised from being heard. Algorithms inadvertently block access to health for the most disadvantaged groups in our society, leaving A&E the only viable option. A 2021 Red Cross report concluded that high-intensity A&E use is closely linked with wider inequalities and deprivation.[31] How do services accommodate the digital divide? Attrition and non-attendance are factors that have to be considered in the provision of services for users with high distress levels and chaotic lives. It may be that as with consultations, a hybrid approach is needed to ensure that patients who need or want to can book appointments in person or by telephone without needing to answer screening questions first; or at least that the screening questions are few in number, open and encourage narrative (e.g. 'What has been happening?'; 'What do you need?'; 'Who would you like to see?'; and 'Would you like a face to face or telephone appointment?') Reception staff must be available to help people who can't fill in the forms themselves.

Culture and Identity – A Relational View

It is unrealistic to expect individuals to practise in a way that prioritizes relationships and person-centred care in contexts which discourage this approach. The culture of the practice affects the consultation styles of its practitioners. Importantly, culture is not fixed, but is dependent on the interactions that take place over time amongst staff members, between staff and patients, and with external bodies such as the CQC and NHS England. In this way, the target-driven, risk-averse and aloof culture of these organizations directly influences the culture of individual general practice teams. Practice cultures generate implicit rules for the clinicians working within them.[32,33] So, for example, in a practice with top-down leadership where the main drivers are financial or performative, consultations are likely to be shorter and more focused on data capture, at the expense of trying to understand the lived experience of the patient. In a similar vein, organizations which respond to issues of patient safety by expanding checklists, inadvertently promote a tick-box culture, where the box is more important than the meaning behind it. This is in contrast to organizations in which members of staff are encouraged to have open discussions about (and preferably with) patients, that focus not only on the biomedical but also on the meaning of the illness for the patient, the emotional impact on the practitioner, and the psychological effect on the patient of their interactions with the healthcare system. Reeve highlights the importance of a learning culture in her 2022 report to the UK Parliamentary Committee.

Protocol, patient safety, and output are the Father, Son, and Holy Spirit of the modern NHS church. These concepts are untouchable and incontestable. But it is we, the medical and nursing professions who define patient safety in the end – it is a medical construct. Think back to the 92-year-old lady with a fast pulse who turned out to be suffering from a broken heart because of the loss of her partner to dementia. Patient safety, output, and protocol dictate that she should have been sent to hospital. We argue that this improves the safety of the *clinician* – in terms of not being criticized for making maverick decisions, but actually worsens the safety of the patient by sending her a long way away to have unnecessary investigations which will ultimately have no bearing on the quality or quantity of her life. The automatization of access to unscheduled care via NHS 111 (see 'Waiting to Connect') reflects the new way of working. If taken to the extreme, the algorithm, like HAL in *2001 Space Odyssey*, should bypass the primary care doctor altogether to maximize 'efficiency' and automatically arrange an ambulance for anyone with a fast pulse without any option of being overridden; and then efficiency could be measured in terms of the time taken to get to hospital and to be assessed. Waiting times through the cascade of patient flow are already key performance parameters. But life is not suited to a flowchart and excluding narrative inevitably makes services less efficient – and ironically, often less safe too (see 'Waiting to Connect'). Chatbots have not been developed to a level which allows them to interpret stories in any meaningful way. Therefore, we still need humans who have the time, willingness, agency, and skill to interpret and listen.

It should be attentiveness, compassion, and accountability rather than protocol, patient safety, and output that sit at the apogee of healthcare services and shape them. We want a service in which these attributes are valued and nurtured and where the approach is overarchingly relational. My (Rupal's) niece recently had a kidney operation, from which she awoke in a great deal of pain. The memory of the nurse who gently gave her a bed bath whilst singing a hymn to her was the most healing part of her post-operative care. If this singing episode came to light, the nurse would not be rewarded, but might instead be criticized for spending too long with one patient, for singing (thus increasing the risk of COVID-19 transmission) and for her choice of a Christian hymn. She will not get a merit award, only a slap on the wrist or reprimand for bringing religion to her act of care. The configuration of the reward system we have is what we have chosen; it doesn't have to be this way. It matters because it directly influences the behaviour of people working within the healthcare system. Reward, not punishment should be given to those who go the extra mile, who take emotional risks, and who privilege relational care. Motives are important. A system is needed in which health workers are permitted to do the right thing, even if this means not doing things 'right'. It is the spirit vs. the letter of the law.

In summary:

- Algorithms which determine access to healthcare do so by using disease categorization (which as we have seen are artificial and potentially misleading, inaccurate, or even harmful) and ignoring biography and nuance. This can render the patient experience frustrating, turbulent and ultimately inefficient.
- Focused attention with good intention is a better measure of quality of care than many others we use. The interaction is as important as the intervention. The presence of too many targets crowds out attention so that it becomes a neglected and untenable proposition.
- Relationships are the cornerstone of decent healthcare, and their absence creates a space in which bureaucracy assumes an unwarranted prominence. That's why continuity is important. Good relationships within teams and between the practice team and its patient population should be given the highest prominence in quality inspections. Emotional engagement should be validated instead of being discouraged.
- Illness narratives do not lend themselves to measurement. Healing is not synonymous with 'sorting and fixing'; it requires imagination and the mobilization of humanity. 'What happened to you?', 'What do you need?', 'What matters to you?' These are the questions we should be asking.
- Guidelines are not tramlines. Clinicians working in primary care need the skills to infer the benefit of medical intervention for their individual patients, taking into account explicit and implicit harm.

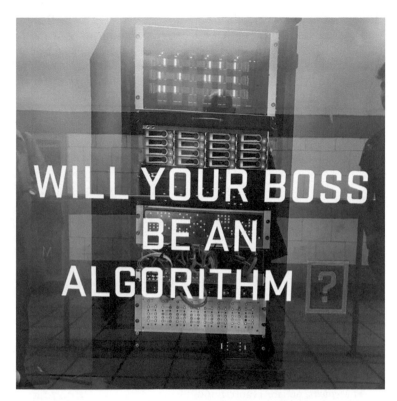

FIGURE C.2: 'Will your boss be an algorithm?' Photograph taken from V&A exhibition advert for 'The future starts here'. Jens Foell, 2018.

- Algorithm, protocol, and regulation are a means to an end – the end being accountability, effective healthcare, protection of the vulnerable, and prevention of abuse. Unlike HAL, they should not have a life of their own beyond this. As things stand, the rules are enshrined in templates and governance structures which are as difficult to change as religious texts, when they should be adaptive and responsive to feedback.

In the end, guidelines, protocols, and ways of checking performance should function as stabilizers to balance healthcare workers. They should not take the place of the cyclist. Don Berwick

217

describes three eras of medicine.[34] Era 1 corresponds to the Doctor and the Doll, the era of unchallenged medical authority. Era 2 is the one in which we find ourselves now; where scrutiny, measurement, accountability, and incentivization predominate. But there is potential for a third era, a moral era that rejects both protectionism and reductionism. It is what we have argued for in this book.

Notes

1. 'NHS Long Term Plan', 2019, accessed December 11, 2022, https://www.longtermplan.nhs.uk/.

2. Department of Health and Social Care, *The NHS Constitution for England*, 2021, accessed January 10, 2023, https://www.gov.uk/government/publications/the-nhs-constitution-for-england/the-nhs-constitution-for-england.

3. S. Harrison, 'Street-Level Bureaucracy and Professionalism in Health Services', in *Understanding Street Level Bureaucracy*, edited by M. Hill, A. Buffat, and P. Hupe (Bristol: Policy Press, 2016).

4. Patrick Brown and Michael Calnan, 'The Risks of Managing Uncertainty: The Limitations of Governance and Choice, and the Potential for Trust', *Social Policy and Society* 9, no. 1 (2010): 13–24.

5. Denis Pereira Gray, Philip Evans, Kieran Sweeney, Pamela Lings, David Seamark, Clare Seamark, Michael Dixon, and Nicholas Bradley, 'Towards a Theory of Continuity of Care', *Journal of the Royal Society of Medicine* 96, no. 4 (2003): 160–66.

6. Victoria Tzortziou Brown, Simon Gregory, and Denis Pereira Gray, 'The Power of Personal Care: The Value of the Patient–GP Consultation', *British Journal of General Practice* 70, no. 701 (2020): 596–97.

7. Christopher Dowrick, *Person-Centred Primary Care: Searching for the Self* (London: Routledge, 2017).

8. Rupal Shah, Sanjiv Ahluwalia, and John Spicer, 'A Crisis of Identity: What is the Essence of General Practice?', *British Journal of General Practice* 47 (2021): 246–47.

9. Daniel J. Martin, John P. Garske, and M. Katherine Davis, 'Relation of the Therapeutic Alliance with Outcome and Other Variables: A Meta-Analytic Review', *Journal of Consulting and Clinical Psychology* 68, no. 3 (2000): 438.

10. Hogne Sandvik, Øystein Hetlevik, Jesper Blinkenberg, and Steinar Hunskaar, 'Continuity in General Practice as Predictor of Mortality,

Acute Hospitalisation, and Use of Out-of-Hours Care: A Registry-Based Observational Study in Norway', *British Journal of General Practice* 72, no. 715 (2022): e84–e90.

11. Royal College of General Practitioners, 'RCGP Response to Comments on "Uberisation" of General Practice', 2022, accessed January 10, 2023, https://www.rcgp.org.uk/News/Uberisation-of-GP-services.

12. J. Michael McWilliams, 'Professionalism Revealed: Rethinking Quality Improvement in the Wake of a Pandemic', *NEJM Catalyst Innovations in Care Delivery* 1, no. 5 (2020): 1–17.

13. Lisa Rosenbaum, 'Peers, Professionalism, and Improvement – Reframing the Quality Question', *New England Journal of Medicine* 386 (2022): 1850–54.

14. Gregor I. Smith, Stewart W. Mercer, John C. M. Gillies, and Alan McDevitt, 'Improving Together: A New Quality Framework for GP Clusters in Scotland', *British Journal of General Practice* 67 (2017): 294–95.

15. Ellen Stewart, Eddie Donaghy, Bruce Guthrie, David Henderson, Huayi Huang, Martyn Pickersgill, Harry H. X. Wang, and Stewart Mercer, 'Transforming Primary Care in Scotland: A Critical Policy Analysis', *British Journal of General Practice* 72, no. 719 (2022): 292–94.

16. Adam Lent, Grace Pollard, and Jessica Studdert, 'A Community-Powered NHS: Making Prevention a Reality', *New Local*, 2022.

17. S. Weil, 'Reflections on the Right Use of School Studies', in *Simone Weil: An Anthology*, ed. S. Miles (London: Penguin, 2003).

18. Elin Martinsen, 'Harm in the Absence of Care: Towards a Medical Ethics that Cares', *Nursing Ethics* 18, no. 2 (2011): 174–83.

19. H. I. Lief and R. C. Fox, 'Training for "Detached Concern" in Medical Students', in *The Psychological Basis of Medical Practice*, ed. V. F. Lief, H. I. Lief, and N. R. Lief (New York: Harper & Row, 1963).

20. John Berger and Jean Mohr, *A Fortunate Man*, 1st ed. (Edinburgh: Canongate, 1967).

21. Johanna Spiers, Marta Buszewicz, Carolyn Chew-Graham, Clare Gerada, David Kessler, Nick Leggett, Chris Manning, et al., 'Who Cares for the Clinicians? The Mental Health Crisis in the GP Workforce', *British Journal of General Practice* 66 (2016): 344–45.

22. Rupal Shah, Robert Clarke, Sanjiv Ahluwalia, and John Launer, 'Finding Meaning in the Hidden Curriculum – The Use of the Hermeneutic Window in Medical Education', *Education for Primary Care* 33 (2022): 1–5.

23. Amanda Lee Roze des Ordons, Janet Margaret de Groot, Tom Rosenal, Nazia Viceer, and Lara Nixon, 'How Clinicians Integrate Humanism in Their Clinical Workplace—"Just Trying to Put Myself in Their Human Being Shoes"', *Perspectives on Medical Education* 7, no. 5 (2018): 318–24.

24. David Zigmond, 'Human Contact: Do We Need It in Medical Practice?', *British Journal of General Practice* 71, no. 710 (2021): 412–13, https://doi.org/10.3399/bjgp21X716933, https://bjgp.org/content/bjgp/71/710/412.full.pdf.

25. Iona Heath and John Berger, *Matters of Life and Death: Key Writings* (London: Routledge, 2018).

26. Stewart W. Mercer, Alex McConnachie, Margaret Maxwell, David Heaney, and Graham C. M. Watt, 'Relevance and Practical Use of the Consultation and Relational Empathy (CARE) Measure in General Practice', *Family Practice* 22, no. 3 (2005): 328–34.

27. Anita Ramsetty and Cristin Adams, 'Impact of the Digital Divide in the Age of COVID-19', *Journal of the American Medical Informatics Association* 27, no. 7 (2020): 1147–48.

28. 'Written evidence submitted by Professor Joanne Reeve (FGP0218)', 2022, accessed May 28, 2022, https://committees.parliament.uk/writtenevidence/41736/html/.

29. Michael Eraut, *Developing Professional Knowledge and Competence* (London: Psychology Press, 1994).

30. 'The Future of Healthcare', Department of Health and Social Care, 2020, https://www.gov.uk/government/speeches/the-future-of-healthcare.

31. British Red Cross, 'Nowhere Else to Turn: Exploring High Intensity Use of Accident and Emergency Services', *A Summary Report 2021* (2021).

32. John Spicer, Sanjiv Ahluwalia, and Rupal Shah, 'Moral Flux in Primary Care: The Effect of Complexity', *Journal of Medical Ethics* 47, no. 2 (2021): 86–89.

33. Rupal Shah, Robert Clarke, Sanjiv Ahluwalia, and John Launer, 'Finding Meaning in the Consultation: Introducing the Hermeneutic Window', *British Journal of General Practice* 70, no. 699 (2020): 502–03.

34. Donald M. Berwick, 'Era 3 for Medicine and Health Care', *JAMA* 315, no. 13 (2016): 1329–30.

Bibliography

Alison, Emily, and Laurence Alison. *Rapport: The Four Ways to Read People*. London: Random House, 2020.

Anonymous Dominican Friar. *Ars Moriendi*. Oxford Polonsky Foundation, Bodleian Library, 1415.

Armstrong, David. 'Actors, Patients and Agency: A Recent History.' *Sociology of Health & Illness* 36, no. 2 (2014): 163–74. https://doi.org/10.1111/1467-9566.12100.

Armstrong, David. 'The Rise of Surveillance Medicine.' *Sociology of Health & Illness* 17, no. 3 (1995): 393–404. https://doi.org/10.1111/1467-9566.ep10933329.

Armstrong, David. 'Professionalism, Indeterminacy and the Ebm Project.' *BioSocieties* 2, no. 1 (2007): 73–84. https://doi.org/10.1017/S1745855207005066.

Bakewell, Joan. 'We Need to Talk About Death.' *BBC Radio* 4, 2017.

Bambra, Clare I. 'Incapacity Benefit Reform and the Politics of Ill Health.' *BMJ* 337 (2008): a1452. https://doi.org/10.1136/bmj.a1452.

Barrett, Lisa Feldman. *How Emotions Are Made: The Secret Life of the Brain*. London: Pan Macmillan, 2017.

Bentham, Jeremy. *Introduction to the Principles of Morals and Legislation. A New Edition, corrected by the Author. Reprinted edition.* Carmel: Liberty Fund, 1823.

Berger, John, and Jean Mohr. *A Fortunate Man*. 1st ed. Edinburgh: Canongate, 1967.

Berwick, Donald M. 'Era 3 for Medicine and Health Care.' *Jama* 315, no. 13 (2016): 1329–30. https://doi.org/10.1001/jama.2016.1509.

Blythe, Jacob A., and Farr A. Curlin. '"Just Do Your Job": Technology, Bureaucracy, and the Eclipse of Conscience in Contemporary Medicine.' *Theoretical Medicine and Bioethics* 39, no. 6 (2018): 431–52. https://doi.org/10.1007/s11017-018-9474-8.

Bourke, Joanna. *The Story of Pain: From Prayer to Painkillers*. London: Springer, 2017.

Bowker, Geoffrey C., and Susan Leigh Star. *Sorting Things Out: Classification and Its Consequences*. Cambridge: MIT Press, 2000.

British Red Cross. 'Nowhere Else to Turn: Exploring High Intensity Use of Accident and Emergency Services.' www.redcross.org.uk. November 2021. https://www.redcross.org.uk/about-us/what-we-do/we-speak-up-for-change/exploring-the-high-intensity-use-of-accident-and-emergency-services.

Brown, Brian, Paul Crawford, and Ronald Carter. *Evidence-Based Health Communication*. London: McGraw-Hill Education, 2006.

Brown, Patrick, and Michael Calnan. 'The Risks of Managing Uncertainty: The Limitations of Governance and Choice, and the Potential for Trust.' *Social Policy and Society* 9, no. 1 (2010): 13–24. https://doi.org/10.1017/S1474746409990169.

Brown, Victoria Tzortziou, Simon Gregory, and Denis Pereira Gray. 'The Power of Personal Care: The Value of the Patient–GP Consultation.' *British Journal of General Practice* 70, no. 701 (2020): 596–97. https://doi.org/10.3399/bjgp20X713717.

Bub, B. 'The Patient's Lament: Hidden Key to Effective Communication: How to Recognise and Transform.' *Medical Humanities* 30, no. 2 (2004): 63–69. https://doi.org.10.1136/jmh.2004.000164.

Carel, Havi. 'Can I Be Ill and Happy?' *Philosophia* 35, no. 2 (2007): 95–110. https://doi.org/10.1007/s11406-007-9085-5.

Carel, Havi. 'Phenomenology as a Resource for Patients.' *The Journal of Medicine and Philosophy: A Forum for Bioethics and Philosophy of Medicine* 37, no. 2 (2012): 96–113. https://doi.org/10.1093/jmp/jhs008.

Carel, Havi. 'The Philosophical Role of Illness.' *Metaphilosophy* 45, no. 1 (2014): 20–40. https://doi.org/10.1093/acprof:oso/9780199669653.003.0010.

Carel, Havi, and Ian James Kidd. 'Epistemic Injustice in Healthcare: A Philosophical Analysis.' *Medicine, Health Care and Philosophy* 17, no. 4 (2014): 529–40. https://doi.org/10.1007/s11019-014-9560-2.

Carville, Serena, Margaret Constanti, Nick Kosky, Cathy Stannard, and Colin Wilkinson. 'Chronic Pain (Primary and Secondary) in Over 16s: Summary of NICE Guidance.' *BMJ* 373 (April 2021). https://doi.org/10.1136/bmj.n895.

Cassell, Eric J. *The Nature of Healing: The Modern Practice of Medicine*. Oxford: Oxford University Press, 2012.

Checkland, Kath, Stephen Harrison, Ruth McDonald, Suzanne Grant, Stephen Campbell, and Bruce Guthrie. 'Biomedicine, Holism and General

Medical Practice: Responses to the 2004 General Practitioner Contract.' *Sociology of Health & Illness* 30, no. 5 (2008): 788–803. https://doi. org/10.1111/j.1467-9566.2008.01081.x.

Cluff, L. E., and R. H. Binstock. 'Introduction.' In *The Lost Art of Caring: A Challenge to Health Professionals, Families, Communities, and Society*, 1–7. Baltimore: Johns Hopkins University Press, 2001.

Cochrane, Archibald Leman. *Effectiveness and Efficiency: Random Reflections on Health Services*. London: Nuffield Trust, 1972.

Cocksedge, Simon, Rebecca Greenfield, G. Kelly Nugent, and Carolyn Chew-Graham. 'Holding Relationships in Primary Care: A Qualitative Exploration of Doctors' and Patients' Perceptions.' *British Journal of General Practice* 61, no. 589 (2011): e484–e91. https://doi.org/10.3399/ bjgp11X588457.

Collings, Joseph S. 'General Practice in England Today. A Reconnaissance.' *The Lancet* (1950): 555–85. https://doi.org/10.1016/S0140-6736(50)90473-9.

Cox, Caitríona, and Zoë Fritz. 'Presenting Complaint: Use of Language That Disempowers Patients.' *BMJ* 377 (2022): e066720. https://doi. org/10.1136/bmj-2021-066720.

Crawford, Paul, and Brian Brown. 'Fast Healthcare: Brief Communication, Traps and Opportunities.' *Patient Education and Counselling* 82, no. 1 (2011): 3–10. https://doi.org/10.1016/j.pec.2010.02.016.

Department of Health and Social Care. 'The Future of Healthcare.' www. org.uk. Updated July 30, 2020. https://www.gov.uk/government/ speeches/the-future-of-healthcare.

Department of Health and Social Care. 'The NHS Constitution for England.' www.gov.uk. Updated January 1, 2021. https://www.gov. uk/government/publications/the-nhs-constitution-for-england/ the-nhs-constitution-for-england.

Donabedian, Avedis. 'Evaluating the Quality of Medical Care.' *The Milbank Quarterly* 44, no. 3 (1966): 166–206. https://doi. org/10.1111/j.1468-0009.2005.00397.x.

Dosa, David M. 'A Day in the Life of Oscar the Cat.' *New England Journal of Medicine* 357, no. 4 (2007): 328. https://doi.org/10.1056/ NEJMp078108.

Doughty, Caitlin. *From Here to Eternity: Travelling the World to Find the Good Death*. London: Hachette UK, 2017.

Dowrick, Christopher. *Beyond Depression: A New Approach to Understanding and Management*. Oxford: Oxford University Press, 2009.

Dowrick, Christopher. *Person-Centred Primary Care: Searching for the Self*. London: Routledge, 2017.

Eraut, Michael. *Developing Professional Knowledge and Competence*. London: Routledge, 1994.

Foell, Jens. 'The Threshold That Connects and Separates, Becoming and Being a Doctor. How Do 5th and 6th Year Medical Students at Imperial College (London) Experience and Manage Uncertainty in Clinical Practice?' *Master of Education, Imperial College London*, 2020.

Freeman, Joshua. 'Towards a Definition of Holism.' *British Journal of General Practice* 55, no. 511 (2005): 154–55. https://pubmed.ncbi.nlm.nih.gov/15720949/.

Fricker, Miranda. *Epistemic Injustice: Power and the Ethics of Knowing*. *Oxford*: Oxford University Press, 2007.

Gabbay, John, and Andrée le May. 'Mindlines: Making Sense of Evidence in Practice.' *British Journal of General Practice* 66 (2016): 402–03. https://doi.org/10.3399/bjgp16X686221.

Galasiński, Dariusz. 'On Medical We.' *Dariusz Galasiński*. December 16, 2017. https://dariuszgalasinski.com/2017/12/16/we/.

General Medical Council. *Ethical Guidance*. London: General Medical Guidance, 2022.

Gray, Denis Pereira, Philip Evans, Kieran Sweeney, Pamela Lings, David Seamark, Clare Seamark, Michael Dixon, and Nicholas Bradley. 'Towards a Theory of Continuity of Care.' *Journal of the Royal Society of Medicine* 96, no. 4 (2003): 160–66. https://doi.org/10.1258/jrsm.96.4.160.

Greenhalgh, Trisha, Jeremy Howick, and Neal Maskrey. 'Evidence Based Medicine: A Movement in Crisis?' *BMJ* 348 (2014): g3725. https://doi.org/10.1136/bmj.g3725.

Grob, Gerald N. 'The Rise of Fibromyalgia in 20th-Century America.' *Perspectives in Biology and Medicine* 54, no. 4 (2011): 417–37. https://doi.org/10.1353/pbm.2011.0044.

Hafferty, Frederic W., and Dana Levinson. 'Moving Beyond Nostalgia and Motives: Towards a Complexity Science View of Medical Professionalism.' *Perspectives in Biology and Medicine* 51, no. 4 (2008): 599–615. https://doi.org/10.1353/pbm.0.0044.

Halpern, Jodi. *From Detached Concern to Empathy: Humanizing Medical Practice*. Oxford: Oxford University Press, 2001.

Harrison, S. 'Street-Level Bureaucracy and Professionalism in Health Services.' In *Understanding Street Level Bureaucracy*, edited by Peter Hupe, Michael Hill, and Aurélien Buffat, 61–78. Bristol: Policy Press, 2016.

Harrison, Stephen, Michael Moran, and Bruce Wood. 'Policy Emergence and Policy Convergence: The Case of "Scientific-Bureaucratic Medicine" in the United States and United Kingdom.' *The British Journal of Politics and International Relations* 4, no. 1 (2002): 1–24. https://doi.org/10.1111/1467-856X.410

Harrison, Stephen, and Ruth McDonald. 'Science, Consumerism and Bureaucracy: New Legitimations of Medical Professionalism.' *International Journal of Public Sector Management* 16, no. 2 (2003): 110–21. https://doi.org/10.1108/09513550310467966.

Hart, Julian Tudor. 'The Inverse Care Law.' *Lancet* 297, no. 7696 (1971): 405–12. https://doi.org/10.1016/S0140-6736(71)92410-X

Hart, Julian Tudor. *The Political Economy of Health Care: A Clinical Perspective*. Bristol: Policy Press, 2006.

Heath, Iona, and John Berger. *Matters of Life and Death: Key Writings*. London: Routledge, 2018.

Hobbes, Thomas, and Marshall Missner. *Thomas Hobbes: Leviathan*. London: Routledge, 2016.

Hommerberg, Charlotte, Anna W. Gustafsson, and Anna Sandgren. 'Battle, Journey, Imprisonment and Burden: Patterns of Metaphor Use in Blogs About Living with Advanced Cancer.' *BMC Palliative Care* 19, no. 1 (2020): 1–10. https://doi.org/10.1186/s12904-020-00557-6.

House of Lords. 'Bolitho V. City and Hackney Health Authority.' www.parliament.uk. November 13, 1997. https://publications.parliament.uk/pa/ld199798/ldjudgmt/jd971113/bolio1.htm

Hull S., and G. Hull. 'Recovering General Practice from Epistemic Disadvantage.' In *Person-Centred Primary Care*, edited by Christopher Dowrick, 1–23. London: Routledge, 2017.

Iserson, Kenneth V., and John C. Moskop. 'Triage in Medicine, Part I: Concept, History, and Types.' *Annals of Emergency Medicine* 49, no. 3 (2007): 275–81. https://doi.org/10.1016/j.annemergmed.2006.05.019.

Kalanithi, Paul. *When Breath Becomes Air*. London: Random House, 2016.

Kennedy, Catriona, Patricia Brooks-Young, Carol Brunton Gray, Phil Larkin, Michael Connolly, Bodil Wilde-Larsson, Maria Larsson, Tracy Smith, and Susie Chater. 'Diagnosing Dying: An Integrative Literature

Review.' *BMJ Supportive & Palliative Care* 4, no. 3 (2014): 263–70. https://doi.org/10.1136/bmjspcare-2013-000621.

Kneebone, Roger. *Expert: Understanding the Path to Mastery.* London: Penguin, 2020.

Kroezen, Jochem, Davide Ravasi, Innan Sasaki, Monika Żebrowska, and Roy Suddaby. 'Configurations of Craft: Alternative Models for Organizing Work.' *Academy of Management Annals* 15, no. 2 (2021): 502–36. https://doi.org/10.5465/annals.2019.0145.

Kubrick, Stanley, director. *2001: A Space Odyssey.* Metro-Goldwin-Mayer, 1968. 1 hr., 43 min.

Larson, Eric B., and Xin Yao. 'Clinical Empathy as Emotional Labor in the Patient-Physician Relationship.' *JAMA* 293, no. 9 (2005): 1100–06. https://doi.org/10.1001/jama.293.9.1100.

Launer, John. 'A Narrative Approach to Mental Health in General Practice.' *BMJ* 318, no. 7176 (1999): 117–19. https://doi.org/10.1136/bmj.318.7176.117.

Launer, John. 'Against Diagnosis.' *Postgraduate Medical Journal* 97, no. 1143 (2021): 67–68. https://doi.org/10.1136/postgradmedj-2020-139298.

Lee Roze des Ordons, Amanda, Janet Margaret de Groot, Tom Rosenal, Nazia Viceer, and Lara Nixon. 'How Clinicians Integrate Humanism in Their Clinical Workplace: "Just Trying to Put Myself in Their Human Being Shoes".' *Perspectives on Medical Education* 7, no. 5 (2018): 318–24. https://doi.org/10.1007/s40037-018-0455-4.

Lent, Adam, Grace Pollard, and Jessica Studdert. 'A Community Powered NHS. Making Prevention a Reality.' New Local. July 12, 2022. https://www.newlocal.org.uk/publications/community-powered-nhs/.

Lief, H. I., and R. C. Fox. 'Training for "Detached Concern" in Medical Students.' In *The Psychological Basis of Medical Practice*, edited by V. F. Lief, H. I. Lief, and N. R. Lief, 12–35. New York: Harper & Row, 1963.

Lipsky, Michael. *Street-Level Bureaucracy: Dilemmas of the Individual in Public Services.* New York: Russell Sage Foundation, 2010.

London Professional Support Unit. 'The Language of Connection.' Health Education England, April 18, 2022. https://vimeo.com/user4672630/review/651088927/b56728738b.

Maben, Jill, Mary Adams, Riccardo Peccei, Trevor Murrells, and Glenn Robert. '"Poppets and Parcels": The Links between Staff Experience of Work and Acutely Ill Older Peoples' Experience of Hospital Care.'

International Journal of Older People Nursing 7, no. 2 (2012): 83–94.
https://doi.org/10.1111/j.1748-3743.2012.00326.x.

Majority Staff of the Committee on Transportation and Infrastructure.
2020. https://www.congress.gov/event/116th-congress/house-event/
LC65141/text?s=1&r=1.

Malin, André, Lars Borgquist, Mats Foldevi, and Sigvard Mölstad.
'Asking for "Rules of Thumb": A Way to Discover Tacit Knowledge in
General Practice.' *Family Practice* 19, no. 6 (2002): 617–22. https://doi.
org/10.1093/fampra/19.6.617.

Mannix, Kathryn. *Listen: How to Find the Words for Tender
Conversations*. London: Harper Collins, 2021.

Mannix, Kathryn. *With the End in Mind: How to Live and Die Well*.
Glasgow: William Collins, 2018.

Marmot, Michael, et al. *Fair Society, Healthy Lives: The Marmot Review.
Strategic Review of Health Inequalities in England Post-2010*. London:
Institute of Health Equity, 2010.

Martin, Daniel J., John P. Garske, and M. Katherine Davis. 'Relation of the
Therapeutic Alliance with Outcome and Other Variables: A Meta-Analytic
Review.' *Journal of Consulting and Clinical Psychology* 68, no. 3 (2000):
438. https://doi.org/10.1037/0022-006X.68.3.438.

Martinsen, Elin. 'Harm in the Absence of Care: Towards a Medical
Ethics That Cares.' *Nursing Ethics* 18, no. 2 (2011): 174–83. https://doi.
org/10.1177/0969733010392304.

Marya, Rupa, and Raj Patel. *Inflamed: Deep Medicine and the Anatomy of
Injustice*. London: Penguin UK, 2021.

Maslow, A. H. 'A Dynamic Theory of Human Motivation.' In
Understanding Human Motivation, edited by C. L. Stacey & M.
DeMartino, 26–47. Cleveland: Howard Allen Publishers, 1958. https://
doi.org/10.1037/11305-004.

Matthews, Sarah, Philip O'Hare, and Jill Hemmington. *Approved Mental
Health Practice: Essential Themes for Students and Practitioners*.
London: Macmillan International Higher Education, 2014.

McWilliams, J. Michael. 'Professionalism Revealed: Rethinking Quality
Improvement in the Wake of a Pandemic.' *NEJM Catalyst Innovations
in Care Delivery* 1, no. 5 (2020): 1–17. https://doi.org/10.1056/
CAT.20.0226.

Mendenhall, Emily. *Rethinking Diabetes: Entanglements with Trauma,
Poverty, and HIV*. New York: Cornell University Press, 2019.

Mercer, Stewart W., Alex McConnachie, Margaret Maxwell, David Heaney, and Graham CM Watt. 'Relevance and Practical Use of the Consultation and Relational Empathy (Care) Measure in General Practice.' *Family Practice* 22, no. 3 (2005): 328–34. https://doi.org/10.1093/fampra/cmh730.

Mohan, J. 'Post-Fordism and Welfare: An Analysis of Change in the British Health Sector.' *Environment and Planning A* 27, no. 10 (1995): 1555–76. https://doi.org/10.1068/a271555.

Montori, Victor M., and Dominique Allwood. *Careful, Kind Care Is Our Compass out of the Pandemic Fog*. London: British Medical Journal Publishing Group, 2022.

Munro, Eileen. *The Munro Review of Child Protection: Final Report, a Child-Centred System*. Vol. 8062. London: The Stationery Office, 2011.

Nelson, Sioban, and Michael McGillion. 'Expertise or Performance? Questioning the Rhetoric of Contemporary Narrative Use in Nursing.' *Journal of Advanced Nursing* 47, no. 6 (2004): 631–38. https://doi.org/10.1111/j.1365-2648.2004.03151.x.

Neuberger, Julia, C. Guthrie, and D. Aaronovitch. *More Care, Less Pathway: A Review of the Liverpool Care Pathway*. London: Department of Health, 2013.

NHS. 'NHS Long Term Plan.' www.nhs.uk. January 7, 2019. https://www.longtermplan.nhs.uk/.

NICE. 'David Haslam: Getting the Guidance Right.' www.nice.org.uk. 2016. https://www.nice.org.uk/news/feature/david-haslam-getting-the-guidance-right.

NICE. *NICE Clinical Guideline 136. Hypertension Diagnosis and Management in Adults*. UK: NICE, 2022.

O'Carroll, Austin. 'The Triple F**K Syndrome: Medicine and the Systemic Oppression of People Born into Poverty.' *British Journal of General Practice* 72, no. 716 (2022): 120–21. https://doi.org/10.3399/bjgp22X718661.

Ofcom. *Digital Exclusion a Review of Ofcom's Research on Digital Exclusion among Adults in the UK*. London: Ofcom, 2022.

Parker, Ruth F., Emma L. Figures, Charlotte A.M. Paddison, James I.D.M. Matheson, David N. Blane, and John A. Ford. 'Inequalities in General Practice Remote Consultations: A Systematic Review.' *BJGP Open* 5, no. 3 (2021): https://doi.org/10.3399/BJGPO.2021.0040.

Porter, Carly, Jasper Palmier-Claus, Alison Branitsky, Warren Mansell, Helen Warwick, and Filippo Varese. 'Childhood Adversity and Borderline

Personality Disorder: A Meta-Analysis.' *Acta Psychiatrica Scandinavica* 141, no. 1 (2020): 6–20. https://doi.org/10.1111/acps.13118.

Ramsetty, Anita, and Cristin Adams. 'Impact of the Digital Divide in the Age of COVID-19.' *Journal of the American Medical Informatics Association* 27, no. 7 (2020): 1147–48. https://doi.org/10.1093/jamia/ocaa078.

Reeve, Joanne. 'Interpretive Medicine: Supporting Generalism in a Changing Primary Care World.' *Occasional Paper (Royal College of General Practitioners)*, no. 88 (2010): 1. https://pubmed.ncbi.nlm.nih.gov/21805819/.

Robertson, Craig. *The Filing Cabinet: A Vertical History of Information.* Minnesota: University of Minnesota Press, 2021.

Rosenbaum, Lisa. 'Peers, Professionalism, and Improvement – Reframing the Quality Question.' *New England Journal of Medicine* (2021): 1850–54. https://doi.org/10.1056/NEJMms2200978.

Royal College of General Practitioners. 'Rcgp Response to Comments on "Uberisation" of General Practice.' www.rcgp.org.uk. January 10, 2022. https://www.rcgp.org.uk/News/Uberisation-of-GP-services.

Sackett, David L., William M.C. Rosenberg, J.A. Muir Gray, R. Brian Haynes, and W. Scott Richardson. 'Evidence-Based Medicine: What It Is and What It Isn't.' *British Medical Journal* 312 (1996): 71–72. https://doi.org/10.1136/bmj.312.7023.71.

Sandvik, Hogne, Øystein Hetlevik, Jesper Blinkenberg, and Steinar Hunskaar. 'Continuity in General Practice as Predictor of Mortality, Acute Hospitalisation, and Use of Out-of-Hours Care: A Registry-Based Observational Study in Norway.' *British Journal of General Practice* 72, no. 715 (2022): e84–e90. https://doi.org/10.3399/BJGP.2021.0340.

Sassi, Franco. 'Calculating Qalys, Comparing Qaly and Daly Calculations.' *Health Policy and Planning* 21, no. 5 (2006): 402–08. https://doi.org/10.1093/heapol/czl018.

Scambler, G. 'Liberty's Command: Liberal Ideology, the Mixed Economy and the British Welfare State.' In *Mind, State and Society: Social History of Psychiatry and Mental Health in Britain 1960–2010*, edited by George Ikkos, and Nick Bouras, 23–31. Cambridge: Cambridge University Press, 2021.

Schön, Donald A. *Educating the Reflective Practitioner: Toward a New Design for Teaching and Learning in the Professions.* San Francisco: Jossey-Bass, 1987.

Schön, Donald A. *The Reflective Practitioner: How Professionals Think in Action.* London: Routledge, 2017.

Sennett, Richard. *The Craftsman*. New Haven: Yale University Press, 2008.

Series, Lucy. 'Making Sense of Cheshire West.' In *The Legacies of Institutionalisation: Disability, Law and Policy in the 'Deinstitutionalised' Community*, edited by Claire Spivakovsky, Linda Steele, and Penelope Weller. Oxford: Hart Publishing, 2020.

Shah, Rupal, and John Launer. 'Escaping the Scarcity Loop.' *The Lancet* 394, no. 10193 (2019): 112–13. https://doi.org/10.1016/S0140-6736(19)31556-9.

Shah, Rupal, Robert Clarke, Sanjiv Ahluwalia, and John Launer. 'Finding Meaning in the Consultation: Introducing the Hermeneutic Window.' *British Journal of General Practice* 70, no. 699 (2020): 502–03. https://doi.org/10.3399/bjgp20X712865.

Shah, Rupal, Robert Clarke, Sanjiv Ahluwalia, and John Launer. 'Finding Meaning in the Hidden Curriculum – The Use of the Hermeneutic Window in Medical Education.' *Education for Primary Care* (2022): 1–5. https://doi.org/10.1080/14739879.2022.2047112.

Shah, Rupal, Sanjiv Ahluwalia, and John Spicer. 'A Crisis of Identity: What Is the Essence of General Practice?' *British Journal of General Practice* 71, no. 707 (2021): 246–47. https://doi.org/10.3399/bjgp21X715745.

Shapiro, Johanna. 'Illness Narratives: Reliability, Authenticity and the Empathic Witness.' *Institute of Medical Ethics* 37, no. 2 (2011): 68–72. https://doi.org/10.1136/jmh.2011.007328.

Shaw, Sara E., and Rebecca Rosen. 'Fragmentation: A Wicked Problem with an Integrated Solution?' *Journal of Health Services Research & Policy* 18, no. 1 (2013): 61–64. https://doi.org/10.1258/jhsrp.2012.012002.

Shorter, Edward. 'History of the Doctor–Patient-Relationship.' In *Companion Encyclopedia of the History of Medicine*, edited by W. F. Bynum and Roy Porter, 783–800. London: Routledge, 1993.

Smith, Gregor I., Stewart W. Mercer, John C.M. Gillies, and Alan McDevitt. 'Improving Together: A New Quality Framework for GP Clusters in Scotland.' *British Journal of General Practice* 67, no. 660 (2017): 294–95. https://doi.org/10.3399/bjgp17X691601.

Sontag, Susan, and Heywood Hale Broun. *Illness as Metaphor*. New York: Farrar, Straus, 1977.

Spall, Bob, Sue Read, and David Chantry. 'Metaphor: Exploring Its Origins and Therapeutic Use in Death, Dying and Bereavement.' *International Journal of Palliative Nursing* 7, no. 7 (2001): 345–53. https://doi.org/10.12968/ijpn.2001.7.7.9019.

Spicer, John, Sanjiv Ahluwalia, and Rupal Shah. 'Moral Flux in Primary Care: The Effect of Complexity.' *Journal of Medical Ethics* 47, no. 2 (2021): 86–89. https://doi.org/10.1136/medethics-2020-106149.

Spiers, Johanna, et al. 'Who Cares for the Clinicians? The Mental Health Crisis in the GP Workforce.' *British Journal of General Practice* 66, no. 648 (2016): 344–45. https://doi.org/10.3399/bjgp16X685765.

Spruill, Tanya M. 'Chronic Psychosocial Stress and Hypertension.' *Current Hypertension Reports* 12, no. 1 (2010): 10–16. https://doi.org/10.1007/s11906-009-0084-8.

Star, Susan Leigh, and James R. Griesemer. 'Institutional Ecology, Translations' and Boundary Objects: Amateurs and Professionals in Berkeley's Museum of Vertebrate Zoology, 1907–39.' *Social Studies of Science* 19, no. 3 (1989): 387–420. https://doi.org/10.1177/030631289019003001.

Stewart, Ellen, Eddie Donaghy, Bruce Guthrie, David Henderson, Huayi Huang, Martyn Pickersgill, Harry H.X. Wang, and Stewart Mercer. 'Transforming Primary Care in Scotland: A Critical Policy Analysis.' *British Journal of General Practice* 72, no. 719 (2022): 292–94. https://doi.org/10.3399/bjgp22X719765.

Svenaeus, Fredrik. 'Hermeneutics of Medicine in the Wake of Gadamer: The Issue of Phronesis.' *Theoretical Medicine and Bioethics* 24, no. 5 (2003): 407–31. https://doi.org/10.1023/b:meta.0000006935.10835.b2.

Swinglehurst, Deborah, Celia Roberts, and Trisha Greenhalgh. 'Opening up the "Black Box" of the Electronic Patient Record: A Linguistic Ethnographic Study in General Practice.' *Communication & Medicine* 8, no. 1 (2011): 3–15. https://doi.org/10.1558/cam.v8i1.3.

Tate, Andy, and Sanjiv Ahluwalia. 'A Pedagogy of the Particular – Towards Training Capable GPs.' *Education for Primary Care* 30, no. 4 (2019): 198–201. https://doi.org/10.1080/14739879.2019.1613677.

Timmermans, Stefan. *Sudden Death and the Myth of CPR*. Pennsylvania: Temple University Press, 1999.

Timmermans, Stefan, and Steven Epstein. 'A World of Standards but Not a Standard World: Toward a Sociology of Standards and Standardization.' *Annual Review of Sociology* 36, no. 1 (month 2010): 69–89. https://doi.org/10.1146/annurev.soc.012809.102629.

Tonelli, Mark. 'The Philosophical Limits of Evidence-Based Medicine.' *Academic Medicine* 73 (1998): 1234–40. https://doi.org/10.1097/00001888-199812000-00011.

231

Tsoukas, Haridimos. 'The Tyranny of Light: The Temptations and the Paradoxes of the Information Society.' *Futures* 29, no. 9 (1997): 827–43. https://doi.org/10.1016/S0016-3287(97)00035-9.

Tsoukas, Haridimos, and Mary Jo Hatch. 'Complex Thinking, Complex Practice: The Case for a Narrative Approach to Organizational Complexity.' *Human Relations* 54, no. 8 (2001): 979–1013. https://doi.org/10.1177/0018726701548001.

Tudor Hart, J. 'A New Kind of Doctor.' *Journal of the Royal Society of Medicine* 74, no. 12 (1981): 871–83. http://www.ncbi.nlm.nih.gov/pmc/articles/PMC1439454/.

UK Parliament. 'Written Evidence Submitted by Professor Joanne Reeve (Fgp0218).' May 28, 2022. https://committees.parliament.uk/writtenevidence/41736/html/.

Veysey, Sheree *A. Look at the Human Being in Front of You Who's Hurting: Clients with a Borderline Personality Disorder Diagnosis Describe Their Experiences of Discriminatory and Helpful Behaviour from Health Professionals*. New Zealand: Unitec, 2011.

Villadsen, Kaspar, and Ayo Wahlberg. 'The Government of Life: Managing Populations, Health and Scarcity.' *Economy and Society* 44, no. 1 (2015): 1–17. https://doi.org/10.1080/03085147.2014.983831.

Wailoo, Keith. 'Thinking through the Pain.' *Perspectives in Biology and Medicine* 59, no. 2 (2016): 253–62. https://doi.org/10.1353/pbm.2017.0010.

Weil, S. 'Reflections on the Right Use of School *Studies.' In Simone Weil: An Anthology*, edited by S. Miles. London: Penguin, 2003.

Winkler, Mary. 'Doctor and Doll.' *AMA Journal of Ethics* 4, no. 2 (2002): 41–44. https://doi.org/10.1001/virtualmentor.2002.4.2.imhl1-0202.

Wolfe, Frederick, and Brian Walitt. 'Culture, Science and the Changing Nature of Fibromyalgia.' *Nature Reviews Rheumatology* 9, no. 12 (2013): 751–55. https://doi.org/10.1038/nrrheum.2013.96.

Wolfe, Frederick, et al. 'The American College of Rheumatology 1990 Criteria for the Classification of Fibromyalgia.' *Arthritis & Rheumatism: Official Journal of the American College of Rheumatology* 33, no. 2 (1990): 160–72. https://doi.org/10.1002/art.1780330203.

Working Party of the Royal College of Physicians. 'Doctors in Society. Medical Professionalism in a Changing World.' *Clinical Medicine (London, England)* 5, no. 6 Suppl 1 (2005): S5–S40. https://pubmed.ncbi.nlm.nih.gov/16408403/.

Zigmond, David. *The Perils of Industrialised Healthcare*. Sheffield: Centre for Welfare Reform, 2019.

Zigmond, David. 'Human Contact: Do We Need It in Medical Practice?' *British Journal of General Practice* 71, no. 710 (2021): 412–13. https://doi.org/10.3399/bjgp21X716933.

Index

Most of the case studies here are amalgams of GP practice experience (see Prologue). In addition to the usual references the index uses *see* or *see also* to indicate named vignettes reflecting a whole story rather than listing only single symptoms or conditions.